W9-CAA-150

THE HEAVY

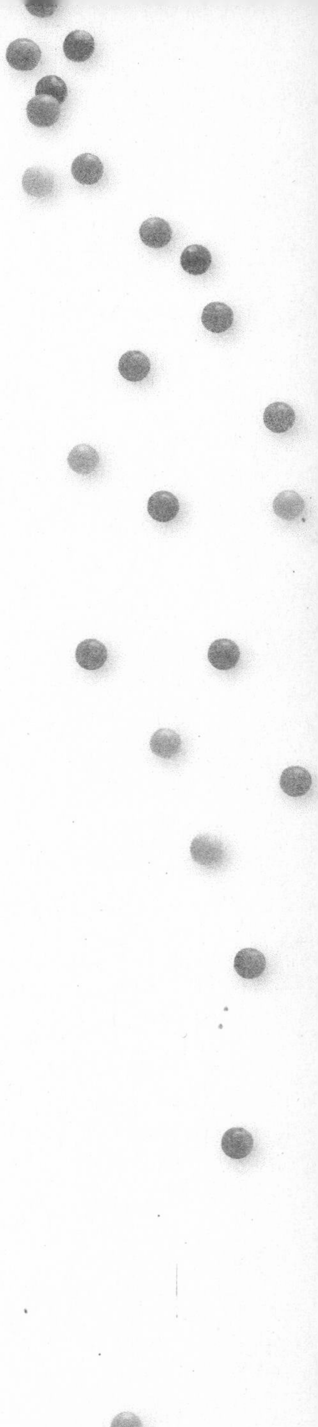

THE HEAVY

A MOTHER, A DAUGHTER, A DIET

A MEMOIR

DARA-LYNN WEISS

BALLANTINE BOOKS
NEW YORK

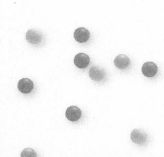

The Heavy is a work on nonfiction. Some names and identifying details have been changed.

Copyright © 2013 by Dara-Lynn Weiss

All rights reserved.

Published in the United States by Ballantine Books,
an imprint of The Random House Publishing Group,
a division of Random House, Inc., New York.

Ballantine and colophon are registered trademarks of Random House, Inc.

ISBN 978-0-345-54134-5
eISBN 978-0-345-54135-2

Printed in the United States of America on acid-free paper

www.ballantinebooks.com

24689753

Book design by Elizabeth A. D. Eno

FOR THE FAM

To paraphrase Tolstoy, all healthy-weight kids are alike, and every overweight child is overweight in his or her own way. What follows is my family's story. Some names—including those of my family members—and identifying details have been changed. Conversations, events, and quotations have been reconstructed to the best of my recollection. Other people involved in the story, including my daughter, Bea, will have their own perspectives on things that likely differ from mine. This book represents my personal experience, and my particular point of view.

—Dara-Lynn Weiss

It was a picture-perfect autumn Saturday. I was walking hand in hand with my daughter, Bea, on a quiet downtown block dotted with cute boutiques and trendy restaurants. Suddenly, something in a store window stopped me dead in my tracks.

"Oh, my God," I muttered breathlessly.

Following my gaze, Bea squeezed my hand tight. We stood still for a minute, taking in the sight before us: row upon row of pastel-hued, buttercream-frosted, expertly decorated cupcakes. Some had cute little flower appliqués. Others bore a playful smattering of sprinkles. They were beautiful.

"Can I have one?" Bea asked.

"No," I answered quickly. A mother's reflex, based on any number of ingrained, "good" parenting tenets: setting limits, the avoidance of sugary processed foods, and protecting her appetite for dinner among them.

"Share one?" she ventured.

Well played, Bea. With those words, she had turned a kid's innocent request into an opportunity for mother/daughter bonding. A chance to connect over our shared love of—obsession with—the indisputably empty calories of cupcakes. Once I was cut in on the deal, I saw the value of the proposition. I grinned at her, and we giddily went inside.

We feasted our eyes on the contents of the display case. Chocolate frosted, red velvet, or classic vanilla? I didn't even have to ask. Classic vanilla, obviously. Where cupcakes are concerned, Bea and I are invariably on the same page, and vanilla is our shared favorite. I bought one.

I took the cupcake from the woman behind the counter, and handed it down to Bea for the first bite. Her big brown eyes widened, and her lips parted in an expectant smile, revealing a prominently missing front tooth. I watched the crumbs collect on her lips as her teeth sank into the thick layer of frosting, and down through the fluffy wall of cake.

My turn: I closed my eyes for a second, savoring the flavor of the delectable treat but more so the exquisite pleasure of spending time with this delightful child. At nearly seven years old, she still thought most of my stupid jokes were funny, and the unselfconscious abandon with which she emitted her hearty laugh made me try all the harder to provoke it. At nearly seven years old, she still generously shared what was on her mind, and I never knew what amazing, hilarious, fascinating thing she might say next. At nearly seven years old, Bea was so easy to please. Why would I begrudge her this simple delight?

If passersby had looked into that cupcake shop window, they would have seen a gleeful little girl enjoying a sweet bite of childhood and a mother happily aglow in the small experience.

If they had children themselves, they might have recognized the kind of ineffable, joyful moment that makes parenting so special.

But our idyll was about to end.

THE HEAVY

CHAPTER 1

The pediatrician walked briskly into the examining room, grabbed the folder from the pocket on the door, and looked at the chart. Bea sat on the examining table in her underwear, her arms crossed over her body.

"She's four foot four and ninety-three pounds," the doctor read. Like all observations she'd made about Bea's health during the previous seven years, this one was made matter-of-factly, almost breezily. But I knew what was coming.

"I need to get some help with her weight," I said, preempting the inevitable reprobation.

"I think it's time," the doctor agreed.

This was a moment I'd dreaded, and now that it had arrived, my heart sank. I'd chided myself about Bea's eating in the months leading to this annual checkup. The pediatrician and I had discussed Bea's escalating weight at our annual appointments for half her life. A year earlier, at the pediatrician's urging, I'd acknowledged that the problem had gone too far, and I'd promised to deal with it.

I'd tried. I'd failed miserably. In the intervening year, my little girl's height had increased normally, while her weight had spiked a stunning twenty-three pounds.

Bea's weight was now equivalent to someone my height (just under five feet four inches tall) weighing 175 pounds. Her blood pressure was 124 over 80, up from 100 over 68 a year before.

There was something about seeing those numbers written into Bea's permanent health record that triggered something primal in me. My reaction was the same as if I'd been told Bea had a potentially fatal allergy, or diabetes. Her weight pattern was no longer a simple parenting hurdle; it was a medical crisis. Something was threatening Bea's health, and I needed to protect her. I needed to figure out how to make the change happen.

If I can look back through time and pinpoint the moment I sat up straight and buckled down, it was then. I knew that I couldn't let my own hang-ups (more on those later), my parenting shortcomings (plenty of those), my fears of screwing Bea up (always, always), my concern about other people's reactions (ingrained, hard to ignore), and the overwhelming difficulty of the task stand in the way of helping Bea become a happy, healthy child. I didn't want my daughter to suffer the health hazards, the emotional pain, the social stigma of being overweight. The buck had to stop there. Even if Bea was only seven years old.

Bea was born an alert, happy, beautiful little girl. She was healthy and met every milestone of physical and intellectual development heralded in the baby books on or before schedule. My only disappointment when she was a baby was that she wasn't a bit chunkier. The first grandchild born to my parents was my niece, at that point the single fattest baby I'd ever seen. And she was scrumptious! Giant eyes with never-ending lashes blinking languidly onto tumescent cheeks. Her sausage-link arms and gargantuan thighs were a total delight. We all wanted to bite her rotund belly, which no shirt seemed able to contain, and on which she rested her chubby hands with Buddha-like calm. Then she grew into a healthy-weight child, and her infant deliciousness was just a cute little footnote. So I'll admit that at first I was the tiniest bit let down that Bea's limbs didn't wrinkle with excess adipose tissue and that her stomach was flat.

Bea had barely been around a year when her brother David was born. They were pretty easy kids. Bea in particular had a maturity and easygoing nature that made my husband, Jeff, and me suspect we were getting off easy in the parenting department. She didn't cry much. She was a reliably good playdate. She talked in full sentences by age two, could read books at age three, and scored in the very top percentiles of every test we subjected her to for the purposes of kindergarten admission.

At home, her unabashed goofiness—often exhibited in improvised dances and high-volume singing—made her little brother laugh so hard he'd nearly choke. She was game for anything and would get excited about even mundane activities such as drugstore shopping or pushing someone's baby in a stroller. Basically, she is a better child than I deserve, a fact my mother jokingly reminds me of constantly.

I was quick to deflect any implication from other people that our parenting had much to do with any of our children's accomplishments. When someone asked what Jeff and I did to get Bea to sit quietly at a dinner table at age two, or for David to learn how to send emails at age three, I would assure them we hadn't "done" anything. "They just came out this way," I'd say.

The differences between David's personality and temperament

and Bea's further disabused me of any notion that our nurture had much to do with how they were inclined to act. My husband and I were, after all, parenting them both the same way (or trying to), and though they were both awesome, there were marked differences.

For example, Bea would instantly learn the words and movements to a song in music class, while David would spend that time tinkering with the technology, figuring out how to work (and blast) the stereo system. Her weakness was bossiness, his was short-temperedness. They were both sensitive and loving, but her affection took the form of a generalized fondness for people, whereas his was a very focused and fiery passion. She preferred playing with boys, while his best friends were girls.

When it came to food, both were good eaters but, again, different. David had clear ideas about what he wanted. A less diplomatic way to say this: he had (has) very precise, narrow tastes in food that, while fortunately incorporating all food groups, were (are still) dauntingly specific. While Bea would happily eat whatever we fed her, David had to have one of the exact vegetables he would tolerate (broccoli, carrots, corn, or Brussels sprouts), one of the two proteins he liked (chicken or beef), and definitely lots of pasta. He would rather starve than eat something he didn't like.

Right or wrong, early on I adopted the theory that kids' essential natures were basically imprinted on them at birth. Sure, somewhere deep in my heart I sometimes took secret credit during proud moments, and also wondered smugly if other kids' misbehavior—a classmate's inability to share, a friend's uncontrollable temper tantrum—were the results of mistakes in their upbringing. Judging someone's parenting is all too easy.

But overall, I believed (still do) that my kids' interests, intellectual capacities, overall health prospects, and dispositions were all in there from the start and couldn't be significantly modified. My husband and I felt that it was our responsibility to help our kids along by constructively molding whomever they naturally were. I couldn't expect David *not* to stand up during music class and blast the stereo. But when he did, did I laugh and praise him for his independent spirit? Did I gently but firmly redirect him back into the circle? Did I grab him and remove him from the class? (I chose the middle option.)

When Bea wasn't sleeping through the night, did we let her cry it out, or did I get up and soothe her back to sleep every time she awakened? (For me it was an inconsistent combination of both.) When David refused to eat the tofu stir-fry the rest of us were enjoying, did I cook him the penne he wanted, or did I give him the choice of eating what we were having or going without dinner? (Mea culpa again: I usually wimped out and made him the pasta.)

I look back on my early new-mom worries with some amusement. Our kids eventually learned to sleep through the night (though as toddlers they were both tough to get to sleep before ten or eleven sometimes), and I trust that one day David's taste buds will wake up. But even as I know that no one misstep will completely make or break our kids, I tend to take each new decision point seriously. Raising a child is, after all, a pretty major responsibility.

Fortunately, Jeff and I generally are of similar mind. We are crazy about Bea and David, but we try to impose limits and order. Not necessarily so well (see cooking pasta to make peace and delayed bedtimes above), but we try.

THE NOT-AT-ALL-TERRIBLE TWOS

When Bea and David started eating actual meals, I did what was expected of modern New York moms and fed my children healthful, well-balanced meals that reflected the latest knowledge of nutrition. Long gone was the USDA-approved food pyramid of the 1970s, which, to my youthful delight, rested heavily on a wide foundation of starchy carbs and included a picture of ice cream in the "dairy" category. Now our carbs have to be whole-grain, and anything with more than five ingredients or an additive your child himself can't pronounce is suspect. You even have to stress out about what kind of water you give him—and it should be in a reusable bottle, but not a plastic one!

Breakfast was not spectacularly nutritious in our home—we ate bagels fairly often, and cereal the rest of the time. But lunch always had a protein in the form of ham or turkey, a piece of fruit, carrot sticks or cucumber slices, and some kind of healthy-seeming organic-ish snack, such as Pirate's Booty or whole-grain pretzels. And never anything other than water to drink.

Dinners consisted of protein (meatballs, chicken cutlets, broiled fish filets), a small side dish of pasta or rice, and vegetables prepared without fat. After-dinner snacks varied from a cheese stick to crackers to a frozen fruit pop to a banana. There was no junk food in our house. At that point, my husband and I had nearly complete control over the kids' diets, and we saw no reason to introduce overtly "bad" foods quite yet.

Parents today can be pretty sanctimonious about what they'll feed to their children, and while I certainly cared about preparing healthful and nutritious meals for my family, in my mind I mocked the moms who were overly concerned with the organic lineage of their kids' food. At a party celebrating Bea's graduation from the two-year-olds program at preschool, I watched as a little girl asked her mom whether she could have an all-natural frozen fruit pop. The mother inspected the ingredient list and said no. I am not sure what the objectionable additive was, but it set a pretty high standard for what that kid was allowed to eat. I think she was permitted a clementine, and that was it. I would never have expressed my feelings to this woman—her kid's eating was her business, as far as I was concerned—but the extent to which she was controlling it seemed absurd.

On the other hand, I also silently disdained the moms who let their kids drink soda or eat fast food. I cringed when I saw fellow mothers on the subway hand their babies a bottle full of some garish pink beverage. And as for parents who had fat kids? Well, the theory that kids are who they are from the start and "just come out that way" went out the window on that one. This was their parents' fault. A lack of discipline or a failure to set limits was at play. These people were either actively feeding their children badly, or passively letting their children feed themselves badly. Either way, logic told me they were to blame, and they were harming their innocent children.

As Bea's weight stayed in the healthy range—maybe even a bit below average for her height—I felt good about the food and activity choices I was making for her, and sometimes looked down on the moms of fat kids the same way I looked down on the moms of poorly behaved kids: maybe the way Bea had turned out was just luck—probably it was just luck—but maybe, just maybe they were doing something wrong, and I was doing something right.

Another thing I was sure we were doing right: Jeff and I did not discuss food and eating in terms of "fattening" or "calories" in front of the children, and I would recoil when anyone else did. Those words had been thrown around casually by parents—

including mine—in the 1970s and 1980s, but now they felt too loaded. Those weren't terms little kids should hear. Since she was a girl and thus, in my mind, more prone to insecurity about her body, I felt Bea needed particular protection from that kind of talk.

At lunch one day in a diner in Queens with Bubby, my grandmother, Bea was enthusiastically chowing down on a piece of my chicken. Bubby gently touched her arm to slow her down.

"Don't eat so fast. You'll eat too much and get fat," Bubby said.

I was horrified. "What the hell, Grandma?" I blurted out. "She's two years old!"

THREE YEARS OLD AND GAINING

It was during the year after Bea turned three that our little girl started to bulk up. With her increased age came additional opportunities for urban exploration and socializing, and with that, exposure to previously unseen cuisines, including junk food.

The first time I ordered Bea her own meal at a restaurant, I was pleasantly taken aback by how voraciously she ate. Fried chicken with peas and potatoes, it was. She pincer-grasped those peas and fed them into her little mouth with tremendous patience, and chewed up more of the chicken than I would have expected for someone so small.

At birthday parties, she sucked juice boxes dry, ate every morsel of the pizza and cake, and enthusiastically consumed whatever candy happened to be in her goody bag. I wasn't bothered by it but did notice that the other little guests didn't do the same. Every block in our neighborhood seemed to feature a cupcake shop, a smoothie joint, a pizza place, or a hot-pretzel vendor, and as we walked, Bea peppered me with entreaties for snacks. Her brother didn't. She loved all foods, including dishes that I found inedibly spicy (chicken with hot peppers) or weird (grilled octopus). She complained constantly of being hungry. She polished off adult-size plates of food. Other kids didn't.

Comparing her growth chart to that of her brother, I see that between the ages of two and six, David gained about five pounds each year, and Bea put on an average of twice that amount. At her checkup when she turned three, her weight was in the 99th percentile. A year earlier, it had been in the 75th-to-90th percentile range. Something was changing.

At a conference with me at Bea's preschool that year, one of her teachers gently sounded an alarm about her eating. "She doesn't self-regulate," she noted. In the classroom, there was a snack table, a dress-up area, an art studio, a writing center, a library, a blocks-building section, and a music station. Guess where Bea spent most of her class time? She'd start off at the snack table and stay there long after her classmates had moved on to other activities. Though she would eventually join them, she'd make frequent stops back at the food for additional nibbles throughout the class period.

Ten pounds a year between the ages of three and six is a noticeable rate of weight gain. At first we saw this merely as a transition from being a slim toddler to being a slightly chunky one. There were other kids who, like her, were carrying around a bit of baby fat. It was sort of cute. Definitely not a big deal.

We also didn't really spend a lot of time worrying about it because, frankly, we were too busy enjoying other aspects of Bea and David. Since they were both healthy, we paid much more attention to their emotional development than their weight.

CONCERN AT FOUR

Bea grew bigger still. She occasionally skipped entire clothing sizes. Jeff pointed out that the size-5 wardrobe I'd been dressing her in when she was four was unbecomingly tight. By the time I brought home a bunch of size-6 replacements, it was too late: she'd outgrown them, too. By the end of that year, she was wearing clothes meant for eight-year-olds. We started having to shorten the legs of jeans meant for much older (and taller) girls so they'd fit her.

I realized this was one of those situations where our response to her behavior, rather than the innate behavior she exhibited, was going to be the determining factor in this issue. But, afraid to send her down an unhealthy path of food obsession and body image problems, I kept my mouth shut. If there was any chance that Bea's weight might not end up being an issue for her physically, I didn't want to make it one psychologically.

But aside from the obvious health problems associated with being overweight, I worried about the emotional implications of letting Bea stay heavy. Were we going to let our daughter be the fat kid in the class? Would her schoolmates tease her? Would she start to hate how she looked? Might she be ostracized in the lunchroom or at recess? What if she grew into an obese adult, as half of overweight six- to eleven-year-olds do? Would her social life suffer? Her self-esteem? Her job prospects? Her potential life span?

I wanted Bea to feel good about herself and her body, but was preaching this kind of self-acceptance wrong if she was actually overweight? Should I teach her to be comfortable with a body that the rest of society disdains, that the medical community cautioned against, and that her father and I personally tried to avoid?

I still held out hope that this was a passing phase that wouldn't require any major action on our part. In light of Bea's appetite,

I was careful to make sure the foods she did have access to were nutritious. She could finish a pint of grape tomatoes or an entire small melon for a snack, so I could only imagine what kind of damage she could do to herself if I'd instead handed her Cheetos or Chips Ahoy cookies.

At that point in Bea's childhood, junk food was not unheard of, but it was still pretty rare. I wouldn't have dreamed of giving a four- or five-year-old kid soda. We almost never ate at fast-food restaurants—maybe once or twice a year. I doled out the kids' Halloween candy haul parsimoniously and raised my voice sharply at grandparents who attempted to sneak them an extra share of dessert at a restaurant. Not because of Bea's weight, but because I felt those were good, healthy habits that I should try to instill in my kids at a young age. No crappy food, no overeating, moderation. Obvious.

HOLDING STEADY AT FIVE

When Bea was five and her weight once again barely fell within the confines of the top of the medical chart, her pediatrician still was not overly concerned. She hoped (as I so desperately did) that the problem would work itself out, that Bea would hit some kind of growth spurt that would eliminate the problem naturally. Bea was also tall, so while her weight was in a high percentile, so was her height. Her annual weight gain, while significant, was staying constant year after year. Her problem wasn't getting better, but it also wasn't getting worse.

The pediatrician waved away the need for any major intervention at that time. She urged us to avoid desserts and sugary drinks. But I knew that wasn't the culprit. We fed Bea nutritious food, and she was no less active than lots of kids her age. Though no athlete,

Bea walked around town, played in the playground like everyone else, and took dance class every week. We confirmed that she had no metabolic or other medical problem causing her weight gain. She just plain ate too much.

CONFRONTING REALITY AT SIX

When Bea was a happy, productive first grader, our adult friends began to acknowledge her weight. "You just can't let her eat like that," one outspoken member of our extended family said. "Get rid of all the processed food in your house," advised my co-worker at the time. "You should get her to exercise more," ventured a mom of one of Bea's classmates. Not that we'd asked.

Bea was catching on to the fact that she was starting to look different from other kids.One afternoon, as we were heading out to a family get-together, I found her in my bathroom putting on my lip gloss.

"So people won't look at my belly," she explained.

Her words cut me to the core. I don't like people looking at my belly either, but I'm in my forties. I hadn't even been aware of my stomach as a potential source of shame until I was years older than Bea. To see her feeling embarrassed about her tummy at such a young age seemed like a premature loss of innocence.

Sometimes, as we cuddled in bed or when she'd get dressed, she'd say, "I'm fat." It seemed disingenuous to contradict her, but unthinkable to agree with her. So I'd dodge. "You're beautiful and healthy. You're growing. You don't have to worry about being fat."

But secretly, I was, increasingly, worried. I asked myself how much of my concern over the superficial, physical aspects of her being overweight was a result of my own ego or vanity. Was I afraid she made me look like a bad mother? Did I worry that other moms thought I was overly lax? Unconcerned with her health? Neglectful? Lazy?

On the flip side, if I tried to put a stop to her patterns, would people think I was overreacting and not giving her time to grow out of her heaviness naturally? I didn't know when the "right" time was to declare war on a child's weight, but I thought age six definitely seemed premature. (Apparently not: a college friend who works in the medical community later confided that when she saw my family that year, with my husband's weight at an all-time high and Bea seemingly following in his footsteps, she was worried. She felt our decision to help Bea did not come a moment too soon.)

So, sure, I wondered what other moms thought about me, and how they might judge my actions or inaction. But I was much more concerned about the judgments Bea herself would be subjected to. I wanted to protect her from the problems inherent in growing up as a "fat girl." I knew people were beginning to view her that way—it was impossible not to—and that their associations with that label were almost always negative. It saddened me to think that people were looking at Bea with anything other than the awe and admiration I felt she deserved.

No matter her weight, I could not love Bea more. And when her belly swelled under a bathing suit or peeked out prominently under her pajama top, my only inclination was to want to kiss it. No weight gain or loss was going to change my opinion of her. Yet while I know a fat Bea would be just as amazing as a thinner Bea, I worried about other people regarding her differently, treating her differently because of her weight. I didn't want people thinking of her as the "fat girl" throughout her childhood. Or ever.

CHAPTER 2

In 1984, a trio of female researchers published an article called "Women and Weight: A Normative Discontent." The title reflected their conclusion that for American women, being unhappy about their weight had ceased to be an anomaly and had become the norm.

Things haven't improved since. After conducting a study of women ages twenty-five to forty-five in 2008, Cynthia Bulik of the University of North Carolina Eating Disorders Program found that 10 percent of the women she surveyed qualified as having an eating disorder, while an additional 65 percent exhibited milder, subclinical levels of troubled eating.

Bulik observed, "It is almost expected that a woman—any woman—is dissatisfied with her body and is trying to lose weight." Obviously, there are exceptions. But each year, approximately forty-five million Americans go on a diet. Inevitably, I'm one of them.

It's been that way since I hit puberty, when I became aware of how my body looked and ashamed of the extra weight I was carrying. Prior to that, my relationship to food and my weight had been fairly unremarkable.

CHILDHOOD NUTRITION, 1970S-STYLE

My two sisters and I grew up in a house where food was not a big deal. There was no overt focus on nutrition, but the meals my parents prepared for us were healthful and well-balanced, at least as the world understood balance and the food pyramid thirty years ago. Breakfast was generally a quickly downed bowl of cereal before the school bus came. Sure, we were into Lucky Charms instead of steel-cut oatmeal, and the milk was whole, not skim. But we weren't scarfing down fast-food breakfast sandwiches or "Breakfast Bake Shop" Hostess donuts either. I did try to make the argument that since these greasy or sugary confections were being marketed as a breakfast food, it was only fair for us to consider them as such, but to her credit, our mother didn't buy in.

The lunches we brought to school might include a turkey sandwich and fruit, or a soggy peanut butter and jelly sandwich. Dinners often began with a half grapefruit or a salad and always contained a protein, a starch, and vegetables.

We were chided for eating too quickly or too messily, for not finishing our vegetables, or for tipping our chairs back at the dining table. But we were not pressured much to eat more or eat less. No one had a health or weight problem when we were little, so food was just food.

I developed a sweet tooth at an early age and could generally find something in my house to satisfy it. There might be something as decadent as a box of Devil Dogs on the corner of the kitchen counter or a box of Oreos in the pantry. More often, the choice was between an Entenmann's Walnut Danish Ring—which I strategically cut for myself to get slices that were heavy on the icing, light on the walnuts—or a freezer burn–ravaged carton of Breyers ice cream.

As we grew up, my sisters developed an enthusiasm and respect for food. They enjoyed eating, cooking, and talking about food. But they did not obsess over it. Their weights were generally stable, and they didn't worry about how their bodies looked any more than the average female did.

GROWING UP CHUBBY

I didn't pay attention to my weight until junior high, when I started to get a little heavy.

My weight gain was understandable, given my activity level and how much I ate. A poor athlete and a lazy person, I exercised only when forced or when I felt it behooved me to try to act more "healthy." I preferred to spend my time reading, writing, or watching *Tic-Tac-Dough* on TV.

I loved eating. And more was better. A latchkey child, I made my own after-school snack, and usually cooked up a pizza muffin or two, followed by a Twinkie or two. My real weakness was peanut butter. On toast, with jelly, or straight up on a spoon—I could down a half cup of the stuff within minutes. At 760 calories and 64 grams of fat for that half cup, it was a dangerous relationship.

At dinner, I would often eat until I felt stuffed. I couldn't understand why someone *wouldn't* eat as many pieces as possible of delicious, golden-brown chicken Parmesan with tangy tomato sauce and slightly browned, melting chunks of mozzarella. It was there, it was delicious, I didn't have to pay for it (at least not financially—

the pounds incurred were another story). Later, I'd dig into the RingDings with the same lack of restraint.

I've spent a good number of hours considering whether there was some emotional component to this eating. It's conceivable that loneliness, insecurity, or boredom contributed to my habits. But I truly believe that my overeating was largely due to my love of food and lack of self-control. With minimal supervision in a household with two working parents, and no formal instruction on what constituted appropriately sized meals and snacks, I just followed my appetite, which was expansive, and directed at the worst possible targets: high-sugar, high-fat comfort foods.

I never became extremely fat. I was always able to wear regular sizes, and no doctor ever said my health was at risk because of my weight. But by eighth grade, I was definitely heavy enough that you'd notice it. I was legitimately chunky. Plump. Zaftig. And I hated it.

So I tried to lose the weight by eating as little as possible all day until my willpower gave out. When it did, I had trouble eating normal amounts of food. By age thirteen, I was constantly engaged in the classic dieting conundrum of mind over matter, willpower versus appetite, id against ego.

I tried everything to get my weight down. I set my alarm clock for four-thirty in the morning to go jogging and bike riding before school. That fitness kick lasted two days. I rode my bike to the supermarket and bought a packet of diet pills. The purchase felt thrillingly precocious and transgressive, like buying alcohol while underage, except in this case, no one asked me for ID at checkout. I didn't tell anyone about my stash of capsules, though their existence likely would not have raised eyebrows. During those years, diet pills and other appetite suppressants were hawked on TV at all times of day (I still remember the tag line from a commercial:

"I lost *weight* with Dexatrim, and I feel *great*!"). In my suburban community, they were practically on the same level as antacids. I occasionally popped one before school, in hopes that it would help me with my plan to eat nothing all day. It didn't.

There was lots of educational talk about eating disorders during those years, both at my school and in the media. It was through that outreach that I learned that sometimes girls took laxatives to lose weight. So I tried it. At the supermarket, they were helpfully and suggestively located right next to the diet pills, and even came in a kid-friendly chocolate-bar format. While they did perform as advertised, the severity of the result (and the disgusting flavor of the "chocolate") were such that I didn't do it again.

At my most desperate moment, I took an emetic in order to make myself throw up after a slightly out-of-control eating session. But generally, my efforts to reduce my size were confined to the Sisyphean task of adopting any calorie-reduction regimen I heard about. I undertook the most ridiculous one at a summer program during high school. It promised five pounds of weight loss in exchange for three days of eating only two eggs, an orange, and broiled chicken. On the morning of the fourth day, I fainted in the hallway of my dorm. That episode prompted a visit to the campus counseling office, where I was referred to a therapist in my hometown. I embarked on a short-lived series of sessions with her, which I didn't mind, but which had minimal effect on my behavior.

At my competitive high school in a well-off, high-achieving community, I was hardly the only kid struggling with eating issues. I would say at least half of the girls in my school were dieting in some way. There was a girl in my grade—popular, smart, accomplished, pretty—who had to be hospitalized for anorexia.

Another girl—happy, well adjusted—would coolly saunter to the bathroom to make herself throw up after eating a big lunch.

Awful as it is to admit, I sometimes wished I could be more like these girls. It was almost a sign of maturity to have an extreme weight loss strategy. One was successful enough in her weight loss efforts to have to be hospitalized for it. And the other so seamlessly and effectively integrated her food neuroses into her day that it hardly seemed like a burden to her. I felt I had the worst of all worlds: starving all the time unless I was gorging on food and feeling bad about myself; lacking both the willpower not to eat *and* the level of commitment necessary to purge; thinking about food and weight constantly, yet still being (in my opinion—and that of a few adults who had the audacity to comment on my physique) chubby.

Then, finally, I was ready to try that quaint, mainstream solution to weight loss: a reasonable diet. An offhand but searing comment from the guy who cut my hair—something along the lines of "You're getting heavy. You should lose weight"—prompted me to join Weight Watchers. After a couple of months of dedicated adherence to the program, I'd dropped the ten pounds that had stood between me and a normal weight, and I was delighted.

Except as soon as I went off the diet, my eating habits reverted to the patterns that had made me overweight to begin with. And so I set to work to lose the pounds I'd regained, reverting to the now-familiar cycle of overeating and deprivation. I wasn't heavy anymore, except by my own standards, but my desire to keep the weight off was as fervent as ever.

My relationship with the scale was a close and intimate one, and I would step onto that thing at least once a day. Most of the time, my mood was at least in part determined by what the scale said.

I grew up in an age when the ideal female form was fairly tiny. As a teenager, I worshipped Madonna, and watched as the attractively fleshy body with which she debuted in 1983 morphed, within a few years, to the more ascetic and sinewy appearance we associate with her today. In the ensuing years, the connection between beauty and voluptuousness of any kind grew weaker and weaker until we reached the 1990s, and it was Kate Moss time.

I adored fashion, and glossy magazines helped shape the unrealistic goals I had for my body. I felt there was no point in having cool clothes if you weren't thin enough to look good in them. But that era's catsuits, tube skirts, and midriff-baring tops were not suited for my build. I saw it as an affront to fashion to be as flabby as I was. Fashion's shift toward "curvier" models such as Gisele Bündchen provided little relief, as it merely replaced the ideal of flat-chested skinny women with one of slightly less flat-chested skinny women. Yes, thanks, that is *so* much more attainable.

Like today, people back then complained about the unrealizable ideals girls were supposed to aspire to, and how "no one really looks like" the women in magazines and on TV. But I felt that wasn't true. I went to school and camp with hundreds of upper-middle-class girls from the New York metropolitan area, and let me tell you, most were thin. The kind of accidental, unstudied thin that comes from being young and metabolically lucky. The kind of body and carefree mind-set that, even when I wasn't heavy, forever eluded me.

Even when I succeeded in (temporarily) knocking some weight off, I still didn't like how I looked. But I was also embarrassed by how much I cared about my weight. I considered my focus on my body akin to being obsessed with tanning. So trivial, and an utter waste of time. Sure, I was a good student, participated in a well-rounded slate of extracurricular activities, and had many good friends. But food and my weight always occupied a disproportionately large place in my thoughts.

I did manage, for one fleeting moment, to succeed in getting my weight down to 100.5 pounds (I'd been hoping to reach 100). But generally, I stayed within a few pounds of 115. Which was a completely reasonable and even attractive weight. But on my build, it wasn't "thin," which is what I wanted to be. So I kept fighting nature.

MY SO-CALLED EATING HABITS: THE COLLEGE YEARS

When I left home for college, I happily realized that I'd grown out of my food issues a bit. My focus on my weight became less consuming, and I was not so different from the other women at school. I wasn't thrilled with my body, but I didn't hate it so much anymore, either.

I was also starting to understand that certain things about my appearance were never going to change. No aerobics class was going to reshape my hips. No amount of weight training was going to get rid of the fat padding my inner thighs. To ameliorate my discomfort with my body, I dressed very strategically. I was blessed with calves that even I didn't think were fat. And so I took to wearing thick black tights with a dress or a short skirt and an oversized top. I wore this uniform pretty much every day from the end of high school through my late twenties. I mean *every* day. Ninety-five-degree summer day? Black tights and a skirt. Snowstorm in the dead of winter? Black tights and skirt.

In a way, it was a form of accepting myself. I was working with my flaws, not trying to eradicate them. But I resented these self-imposed limitations. To me, being thin represented freedom. Freedom to wear whatever I wanted. To raise my arm without worrying about pulling my shirt down over my stomach. To lean over without feeling a roll of fat fold around my midsection. To put on a little black dress and head out to a party without having to suck in my gut the whole night. It meant having nothing to hide.

Junior year, I suffered a weight gain of thirty pounds, attributable to a pint-a-day addiction to Häagen-Dazs Chocolate Peanut Butter ice cream. I needed to get that weight off. But I wanted to eat what I liked. And I didn't want to have to exercise much. So I adopted a diet that entailed eating only moderate amounts of my favorite foods, forgoing any superfluous fruits, vegetables, and proteins along the way. I'd have a daily breakfast of some small sugary treat (a slice of pound cake or an ice cream bar), then down an entire box of mac and cheese or a slice or two of pizza for dinner. And I returned to my normal weight.

When I'd spend time with my family, my sisters joked about my eating. One of them would cook a healthful dish while I'd break open a box of cookies, and each of us would mock the other. To me, it was lunacy to pass up a food you loved for one you liked less just because the latter one was more healthful. To them, having an occasional Cinnabon for dinner was bonkers.

My older sister, with amused faux formality, referred to my approach to eating as "the Theory of Food Mass Consumed." Basically, I was challenging the idea that calories matter all that much, and paying no attention to fat versus protein versus carbs (just to orient you, this was still during the era when fat was bad and carbs were good). Instead, I believed weight maintenance was all about the mass of the food you ate.

For example, your egg-white omelet with spinach and my ice cream sundae of similar density and weight were equivalent. If you ate a little bag of carrot sticks and I ate a slightly bigger bag of potato chips, we were pretty much even, even though my meal's calories far outstripped yours. I posed a question to myself: if I could somehow take a pill containing 10,000 calories, would it make me gain three pounds? My guess was no, since its mass was only equivalent to that of a peanut.

I developed the Theory of Food Mass Consumed with a suitable level of irony. But frankly, the medical health-and-nutrition establishment hadn't exactly done much to earn my faith in the decades during which I struggled to figure out what to eat to lose weight. In the 1980s, fat was the villain. In the 1990s, it was carbs. In the 2000s, it was junk food and inactivity. In the 2010s, all charges were leveled against insulin-processed sugars and starches.

Each theory made perfect sense at the time, and I briefly tried to incorporate each into my habits, only to have it debunked. With so many conflicting messages, it's nearly impossible to figure out how to eat. And while the nation has gotten fatter and fatter listening to these experts, I successfully employed my Theory of Food Mass Consumed for many years. So is it ridiculous? Of course. But it worked for me.

DIET AND THE SINGLE GIRL

I maintained my weight in this way through my twenties, although I always pitied myself that I was "dieting." All week I'd deny myself any excess, and then on the weekends, I'd splurge and undo all the progress I'd made. The moment I let myself eat without restraint, my weight headed upward, and come Monday, I'd rein in my consumption in order to bring it back down.

What I didn't realize was that my "diet" was a diet in the true sense of the word: not a temporary weight-loss effort, but a continual, habitual way of eating. If I wanted to maintain my weight, yet eat with abandon several times per week, I was going to have to be on what felt like a "diet" the rest of the time.

Then I got married. To a guy who also struggled with his weight. I found him adorable, attractive, kind, funny, brilliant. And I still do. So what if he had—and has—a belly? I didn't care.

Together, Jeff and I went on various diets, joined a gym, visited a nutritionist. Nothing helped.

BRINGING UP BABIES

Then I got pregnant with Bea. I was excited for many reasons, most of all because I wanted a baby; I was looking forward to being a mother. But a little bit of my joy stemmed from the promise of nine-plus months of pregnancy and the attendant freedom from food guilt and body image shame. Back in the late 1980s, as a seventeen-year-old intern at a Madison Avenue advertising agency, I had watched a pregnant woman in my department hobble in every day, grumpy and frumpy, and feel pangs of jealousy. *She can eat whatever she wants!* I marveled. *She can get enormous, and no one will judge her for it!*

Yes, I know, it's totally pathetic that as a pre-college woman starting her life in the big city, the object of my envy was a decidedly unglamorous, midthirties pregnant media planner. But the idea that I might one day be able to spend nearly a year not having to hold in my stomach was thrilling to me.

My weight gain during that pregnancy was exactly as I had anticipated: swift and significant. I gained sixty pounds before Bea finally made her debut. And just as I was getting around to thinking about losing that weight, when Bea was about four months old, I got pregnant with David. That happy (if surprising) event forestalled any further thoughts of dieting.

After David was born and my body settled down, I joined the army of postpartum moms who turn to Weight Watchers for help losing the leftover baby weight. I stuck to the program devotedly, and attended meetings every week. For five months, my weight went slowly down until I'd lost twenty pounds.

It's a reflection of how far I had come since my twenties that I was genuinely satisfied with my new weight, even though it was higher than any I had tolerated before having children. It didn't hurt that, for the first time in my life, my age had caught up to my body. The physical attributes that to me had seemed sort of pathetic on a teenager—slack stomach, muffin top, cottage cheese butt—were normal for a thirty-five-year-old woman. Plus, my lifestyle no longer involved miniskirts, and the current fashion was for long T-shirts instead of cropped ones, so I was in a good place.

Further evidence of my healthier approach to food and my body was the fact that I didn't fall off the wagon in some dramatic way once I reached my goal weight. I stayed at or near that weight for several years until suddenly, randomly, I lost a few extra pounds without really trying.

I got used to my new, lower weight quickly. When those pounds tried to come back, there was a new solution that had just hit the scene: juice cleanses! Men and women, fat and not, were undertaking these "cleanses," which ranged from fancy six-bottle-a-day delivery services to homemade concoctions of cayenne pepper, maple syrup, and lemon juice. A masochistic penance for overindulgence.

A few days of drinking only juices would bring my weight back down, for like five seconds. At this point Bea was in first grade, and

David was in kindergarten, and they were for the first time aware of what I was eating (or not eating). When they asked what I was drinking from those weird bottles, I tried to extol the nutritional value of the kale-spinach-romaine-cucumber combo I was forcing myself to ingest. But of course, that wasn't really why I was doing it. I didn't care about the "detox" aspect—I was just in it for the weight loss.

Like a get-out-of-jail-free card, the promise of a juice cleanse was allowing me to slip back into yo-yo dieting habits that I thought I'd given up after I'd become a mom. I was disappointed in how I was eating and feeling about my weight. I also didn't like that I was so publicly and stupidly wrestling with these insecurities just as Bea was becoming self-conscious about her own weight. One had to trip over a digital scale to get into my bedroom, and I would grunt in self-disapproval and kick off a juice cleanse when the number it displayed got too high. I wanted Bea to be receiving more positive, less confusing messages about body image and healthy weight maintenance. I knew I was letting her down in that department.

But the fact was: for the prior three decades, I had not attended a party, sat down to a meal, gone to the bathroom, or been physically ill without, on some level, silently calculating how that action would affect my weight. I'd be miserable from the flu, but a little voice inside of me would see the silver lining that the loss of appetite I was suffering meant I might be losing weight.

I recall the day over a decade ago when a slim, cool co-worker of mine came into my office and gruesomely described the food poisoning she'd fallen victim to over the weekend. Then she confessed that as she was vomiting, it had brought her some comfort to realize doing so was probably taking about a pound off her weight. I laughed with relief and recognition, glad that someone else had those thoughts. If only I'd known how many other women shared my experience.

I had avoided addressing Bea's problem for fear of projecting these kinds of thoughts about food and weight onto her, hoping that I could spare her the fate of wasting years disliking and vainly trying to change her body. But the worst-case scenario was not that Bea would end up like me. Distressingly, her situation stood to be much more dire than my own.

You see, I don't come from an overweight family. I've explained how strong a role I believe genetics plays in determining who we turn out to be. So, for example, it's no surprise to me that I'm short—so are my mom and dad, and so were their parents. And in my heart, I knew it was unlikely I would ever really become morbidly obese because of that genetic predisposition.

But the same isn't true of Bea. The same healthy weights that characterize my side of the family can't be said of my husband's side. Jeff loves food as much as I do, but unlike me, he has been overweight or obese all his adult life. His parents and grandparents have struggled with their weight, too. His size, blood pressure, and cholesterol levels are sufficient to require the concern and monitoring of his doctor. Bea has a genetic predisposition for obesity.

Jeff didn't become heavy until his late teen years. Now here Bea was, exhibiting the behaviors and size of an overweight person, and she was only six years old. Further, her world featured far more temptation from food and weight gain pitfalls than had been available even a generation before. More damage could be done.

I had worried that if Bea took after me, she would suffer the physical and emotional ups and downs I had gone through regarding my weight. But I began to realize that Bea was on a much worse trajectory. Issues aside, I'm a healthy woman at a healthy weight. While the occasional peculiarities of my diet weren't causing me serious physical harm, Bea's way of eating was legitimately dangerous. She was on track to spend her life being overweight and battling the problems that come with it: high blood pressure, diabetes, difficulty moving, heart disease, poor self-esteem, social isolation, depression.

With that recognition, I couldn't continue being silent and being absent as a role model any longer. I didn't feel responsible for engendering Bea's problematic relationship with food, but at this point I felt I was definitely enabling its continuation.

As a mother, I try to imbue my kids with self-esteem and instill in them a positive body image despite my own body dissatisfaction. It's a challenge. I had come of age in a time of enormous body-image pressure, and it was hard to shrug all that off in order to set a positive example for my own children. How can a woman who steps on the scale religiously, diets regularly, and won't consider wearing 99 percent of commercially available clothing because she thinks they make her look fat parent an overweight child? I wanted to help Bea get healthy while also passing on sound eating principles and body image positivity, neither of which I possessed myself. In order to navigate with Bea through this issue, I knew I had to change. I had to be better.

CHAPTER 3

If my own history with eating had left any question as to my ill-preparedness to deal with Bea's weight problem, all doubts were erased during the year I tried in vain to help her myself.

It began after Bea's checkup a few weeks after she turned six. Finally acutely aware that Bea ran the risk of turning into the worst possible hybrid of my husband and me in terms of eating habits, body image, and obesity, I promised the pediatrician that I'd address her weight. I tried to institute some new habits. Taking a cue from the widely disseminated professional advice on how to treat childhood obesity, I thought the changes we needed to make would be easy—give her more fruit and whole grains, sneak carrots and spinach into her smoothies, limit screen time, get her up and moving—and the results decisive.

Lack of physical exercise is always one of the factors blamed for why today's kids are overweight. I understand how frustrating it must be for people to look at the epidemic of childhood obesity and to think, *Why aren't these kids just getting more activity?* It is normal to assume, if your child is a healthy weight, that your family's food and activity choices are responsible for that fact, and that if other families did as yours did, their kids would be healthy, too. But the fact is, Bea was no less active than her healthy-weight peers: she took dance class, ran around with her friends during recess and gym at school, and went to the park when weather permitted. But she didn't come close to engaging in the kind of consistent, calorie-burning activity required to make a dent in a child's weight.

Let me start with the easy excuses. My family lives in a small apartment in the city. There's no backyard to run around in, no school teams practicing sports every weekend like my suburban elementary school had. My commitment to help Bea began during a harsh winter, and playground visits were impossible when temperatures were in the twenties. Justifications notwithstanding, I felt that eating adjustments were going to have to carry most of the burden of the lifestyle changes she needed.

We tried portion control—if we got bagels, I'd encourage Bea to eat only a half. As city dwellers in a neighborhood where dining out can be cheaper and quicker than cooking at home, we found ourselves eating lunch or dinner in a restaurant at least once a week. On those occasions, I offered to split an entrée with her. But she rightly complained that it was unfair that only she be subjected to these limitations when her brother and her friends were under no such constraints. There is something demeaning and infantilizing about having your mom lop off half of your burger and grab a big handful of french fries off your plate before you can start eating. Fair enough. So sometimes we shared food, sometimes we didn't.

We tried substituting better foods for the least healthful ones in our repertoire. I grilled the kids' chicken cutlets instead of pan-frying them. I forced David to try whole-wheat pasta instead of the regular kind (he hated it). When someone suggested ice cream, I'd jump in and offer to make fruit-and-yogurt smoothies instead. But we had been eating pretty nutritiously to begin with, so there really weren't many changes to make in that area.

I did notice that when Bea was on a regimented school-year schedule and ate only the food I gave her for breakfast, lunch, and dinner, her weight gain slowed a bit. I could tell by how much her stomach stuck out: similar to my own weight, the stomach was the leading indicator of where the entire body was trending. When her schedule wasn't as structured and she had more free time to eat, her weight went up.

When it came to snack food choices, I was woefully inconsistent. Bea's school bus stop happened to be in front of an Au Bon Pain. On most days we stepped inside to find our after-school snack. Offerings ranged from small cups of watermelon to a 1,000-calorie corn chowder soup in a bread bowl, and I was never sure what to get her. A small tuna sandwich? A cup of chicken noodle soup? They seemed like wholesome choices, but were they more meals than snacks?

Some days I tried to do the right thing and insisted on fruit salad or a single hard-boiled egg. But occasionally I'd give in to her pleas for a square of coffee cake, mainly because I wanted to eat half of it. And every day I wondered, how much should a kid eat after school? And was the answer different if the kid was heavy?

Opportunities for treats on special occasions also elicited irregular responses. When cupcakes came out at a party, sometimes I gave her the go-ahead, and other times I grimaced with disapproval, depending on my mood and my anxiety about her weight that day. And then I might even sneak one (or two) for myself while she wasn't looking. Of course, unpredictability and hypocrisy are not parenting virtues.

Complicating matters was the fact that we were usually with David, who did not share Bea's weight problem. David could have basically whatever he wanted for his after-school snack, from Italian ices to two slices of pizza. If he wanted an extra helping of breakfast or a snack at bedtime, I gave it to him gladly—because he asked for it so rarely, and because he was not overweight. But I had no rhetoric for justifying the double standard when Bea pointed it out.

While Bea never expressed concern about the food she ate, her body's appearance was beginning to bother her. And I desperately wanted to say the right thing in response to the self-deprecating remarks she made about her size. But I had no idea how to respond to a child who complained of being fat if that child was, indeed, overweight.

Now that she was no longer a toddler and her weight problem had persisted for years, I charily decided that, instead of telling her not to worry about it, I should acknowledge the problem and offer help.

So when she called herself fat, I tried a new tactic. "You are beautiful," I said (which, for the record, she is). "Yes, you are a bit overweight. And we can fix that by changing the way you eat. Do you want to do that?"

That conversation led to a discussion about how for her, achieving a healthy weight might mean, for example, eating less pizza.

"But I like pizza!" she replied in mock outrage.

"I know, but having a lot of it can make you overweight. And cupcakes . . . ?"

"Mmmm! *Cupcakes*!"

"Yeah, they're okay once in a while, but I feel like we've been eating them every week, sometimes more."

"Cupcakes are *so good*."

"I know."

"Can I have one now?" she asked.

In my mind, I said, *Yeah, a cupcake sounds pretty good right now.* But instead I answered, "Unfortunately, no."

"I want a cupcake," she sighed.

Me too, I thought, remembering our stolen moments together, sharing our favorite vanilla-frosted cupcake. Those innocent, delicious, spontaneous yeses in a world filled with nos. I didn't want to give them up any more than she did. So things continued as they had.

One comment during that year broke through to me more than the rest. I was sitting down at lunch with an octogenarian friend, a warm, wise man whom I look to as a grandfather figure, even though he is not a blood relation. He'd known Bea and David all their lives but hadn't seen them in a while.

We began catching up. I showed him a recent photo of Bea and David as I described their latest accomplishments.

He squinted at the photo, leaning in to examine it more closely. His smile slackened slightly.

"Is Bea getting heavy?" he asked.

"Um . . . yes," I admitted.

He put the photograph down on the table and fixed me with his gaze. "Don't let her," he admonished.

"What am I supposed to do?" I asked.

"Don't let her," he repeated firmly.

And while on the face of it he was supplying no guidance, he was actually providing a huge directive: it was up to me to stop this problem, which clearly wasn't going away on its own. The words echo in my mind to this day: *Don't let her.*

As for Bea, there was one comment that stuck with her, too. A mean kid in her class took to calling her "Fatty Patty." Not always, not even often, and certainly not with any evidence of originality or wit. But when she related the story to me at home, I was at a loss. The knee-jerk retort "Well, you're *not* fat, so screw him" would have been a lie. Nor did it seem as if I should turn it into a teachable moment and launch into a complex discussion of childhood obesity.

So I just hugged her. And she cried, and it broke my heart. I told her that boy was mean and jokingly promised that I would make him rue the day he ever opened his mouth to her. (He happened to move to Missouri shortly thereafter, never to be seen by us again. That was a happy accident, but to this day I still tell Bea it was my doing and ask whether there are any other classmates she doesn't like who should be "moved to Missouri.")

Another time, a classmate rather blandly noted, "Bea, you have a big belly." Once again, the observation didn't win any points for cleverness, but it hurt Bea's feelings. When she told me about it, I asked how she'd responded. Tears rolled down her rounded cheeks. "I was just so humiliated, I didn't say anything."

Again I drew her close and hugged her tight but was uncertain as to what to say. This kid wasn't even trying to be hurtful; he was just observing a plain fact. Bea's belly was uncommonly large, and kids noticed.

It killed me to hear these stories. But I admit that a tiny part of me wondered if maybe they were useful for motivating us in some way. Being overweight is so blatant, so public, by age six Bea was already having to confront the embarrassment of it. While the potential for future health hazards may have been enough to spur me to action, I wondered if perhaps Bea would be motivated by a desire to be spared the humiliation she was starting to suffer from her peers.

But after the tears had subsided, Bea asserted that these comments, while upsetting, didn't nudge her to try to look different. She was quick to venture that the mean kids would likely just find something else to tease her about, and she's probably right. To her, the insult was hurtful because it was meant to be insulting. The inherent judgment about her weight was less powerful to her.

Over the summer before second grade, Bea went back to the camp she loved from the summer before, which had the distinct disadvantage (to me) of featuring an all-you-can-eat cafeteria. While I'd throw a few pieces of advice at her each day when I dropped her off ("Hey, today's pizza day—only one slice, okay?"), the freedom of making her own lunch choices took its toll.

When Bea returned to school, I redoubled my efforts to control her eating by packing her lunchbox with salads and fruit, which she loved. But for the first time, I didn't see her belly get smaller. Having her take gymnastics class once a week in addition to her usual activity, encouraging more visits to the playground, suggesting we not let dessert be an everyday occurrence, offering to split a burger instead of each of us getting our own—even though I was trying, these changes weren't making a difference.

I began referring to foods as "healthful," "not healthful," or "okay if you don't have too much" as euphemisms for "low-calorie," "fattening," or "something really delicious and fattening that if you share with me won't be so bad for either of us." I was grasping at straws.

I felt incompetent because I had no idea really how much—or what—she was supposed to eat. I didn't know whether to stop feeding her, despite her protests, when I felt she'd had the proper amount, or let her eat a second serving in order to preempt between-meal snacking. Was it hypocritical to consider a slice of pizza a perfectly reasonable snack for David, yet a dangerous one for Bea? Or was my double standard appropriate?

The media provided me with no helpful role models. The only stories I'd heard about childhood struggles with weight—from *Celebrity Fit Club* contestants to reality-show stars—involved insensitive parents who subjected their children to derision and bullying for being fat at age five and are now being blamed for launching the child into an unhealthy relationship with food.

There's also a staple sitcom character, the food-obsessed thin girl (see Monica on *Friends,* Grace on *Will & Grace,* Liz Lemon on *30 Rock,* et al.), who is often given the character detail of having been fat as a kid. Yes, isn't it adorable to see such a skinny woman eat with abandon? And isn't it great that she can do so without being fat, even though she is, according to her character sketch, genetically predisposed to being overweight? It's funny to see a former fat kid stuff her face, assuming she can keep the pounds off through the magic of fiction.

Both of these characterizations bother me—the girl whose parents' handling of her weight caused lifelong problems with self-esteem and eating, and the woman who somehow grew out of her obesity unscathed, transforming into a svelte swan despite her persisting appetite. In the first scenario, the child is made to endure too much pain for her weight problem; in the latter, she gets off too easy.

In the event that a child first needs to reach a healthier weight before it's appropriate to encourage her to accept her body the way it is, I propose that a new role model evolve: one in which a child with an big appetite and the weight to match is parented by someone who intervenes in a productive, healthy manner. Obviously, if I went around belittling Bea about her weight without providing any useful leadership, that likely would not have a positive outcome. But neither would saying nothing and hoping the problem just goes away, as it does on TV.

Given my discomfort with issues of food and weight, silence was the first path I chose. Knowing that I was going to have to open my mouth at some point soon was scary. When our kids were both a healthy weight, it was easy for Jeff and me to pat ourselves on the back for the food and activity choices we were making for them. Now, with Bea overweight, those same decisions had to be called into question. And while at any given moment I wouldn't have hesitated to tell David to stop eating something if I felt it was appropriate, telling Bea the same thing seemed a much more fraught maneuver.

After confronting my failure at that pediatrician appointment when Bea was seven, I refused to let my incompetence, embarrassment, or hesitance be an excuse for letting Bea get heavier and heavier. Helping her was now a medical necessity. If she needed help, so did I.

CHAPTER 4

Just before Bea's seventh birthday, my husband and I received an email from a trusted friend. It was a forward of a newsletter she had received from a mom she knew whose daughter was a client of a pediatrician who specialized in child obesity. "Just in case you're interested," the email began gently, "this friend has really liked this program and felt it wasn't stigmatizing at all—nor does it make kids nuts about food."

I clicked a link in the email over to the nutrition doctor's website, which explained her program and how it uses the metaphor of traffic lights to help kids make good food choices. Green-light foods are encouraged, yellow-light ones require a bit of caution, and red-light ones are reserved for occasional treats. It sounded reassuringly like the Weight Watchers Points system I found so sensible and effective for my own weight management. Food choices are assigned values, and aside from some reasonable nutritional requirements, you could choose your own adventure within your personal food budget.

The nutrition doctor behind this program had literally written the book on pediatric and adolescent weight loss. On Amazon I could see that the slick volume featured colorful charts, sophisticated graphics, and gorgeous food photography. I was impressed.

The most convincing thing was the handful of before and after pictures of kids the doctor had treated. One girl looked remarkably like Bea. Many were of a similar age and weight. Despite the reported epidemic prevalence of overweight and obese children, I had felt quite isolated in my predicament, and it was a relief to see other kids like mine.

The decision about whether to call this doctor—and if so, when—fell to me. Jeff and I discussed Bea's weight problem and agreed we needed to address it, but I had more time to dedicate to it. In order to spend more time with my kids, I'd put my career as a producer of Web and television content on hold a bit and was only employed part-time. My job at that time involved working from home, reviewing footage of cooking shows for a television production company in the morning and taking care of the kids after school. So my schedule was far less demanding than Jeff's, whose job running a nonprofit requires late hours and frequent travel.

In most families I know, one parent takes ultimate responsibility for the day-to-day drudgery of childrearing, and in our family, that parent is me. I wake the kids up in the morning and put them to bed at night. I prepare and serve all their meals. I make sure teeth are brushed, homework is done, baths are taken, shoes are tied, medications are dispensed, and boots are worn on rainy days. I don't mind it. I consider it part of my job description. I'm the heavy. So I knew that a new food regimen, too, was going to be under my jurisdiction.

But Jeff strongly believed that the whole family should be in it together. It shouldn't just be Bea who went to nutrition-doctor appointments and adhered to a new eating plan. It should be all of us. So that Bea wouldn't feel singled out, we were going to present the endeavor as a campaign for healthful family eating, not a Bea-needs-to-lose-weight project. Each of us had some issue that could stand improvement—from Jeff's need to lose weight to David's starch-heavy diet to my juice-cleanse crutch—so we could legitimately argue that we all needed a nutritional makeover.

Thanksgiving was coming, along with both kids' birthdays (which required in-school cupcakes, family dinners on their actual birthdays, and of course the birthday parties themselves), winter break, Christmas parties, Chanukah observances, and New Year's. I wanted to start our new program after the holidays but arranged with the nutrition doctor's office for Jeff and me to meet with her first. He wanted to make sure we liked her and approved of her approach before bringing in the kids.

We arrived for our appointment at the doctor's office on a busy block in midtown Manhattan on an overcast Friday afternoon in December. We sat down with the nutrition doctor, who began by describing the program. It was flexible enough to let kids eat like kids, tailoring food choices to each child's preferences, and allowing for inevitable splurges. Her philosophy was that no child on the program should ever have to decline a piece of birthday cake, or feel left out of a pizza party. The key was to empower the child to make her own decisions within the program's framework.

She explained that at our initial family consultation, each family member would have his or her BMI and other factors evaluated. At the next appointment, we'd receive a breakdown of how many "green lights" (which loosely translated into units of 100 calories) we get at each meal and snack. We'd be given a reference book listing how many "green lights" are in common foods and how to calculate the traffic-light value of any other foods. We would be required to eat a certain amount of fruits and vegetables every day and not to overdo it on unhealthful foods. But within our allocation of traffic lights, we could pretty much put together our own daily menus.

Immediately I thought, *She gets it.* This wasn't a nutritionist who tells you junk food is bad and whole grains are good, or who encourages you to squeeze more fruit into your diet without taking anything else away. This was someone who understands that overweight kids need to eat less.

She explained that there are two kinds of diets: the calorie restriction method, in which you eat any kind of food but limit your quantities (such as the Weight Watchers Points system), and the approach where you don't count calories but limit your food options (such as low-carb diets). She didn't think either system was particularly successful. Her program was a combination: limiting overall calories but also encouraging better food choices. It struck me as the right way for a kid to go about it: nothing was off-limits, but good habits could be instilled in the process of taking weight off.

I loved that she wasn't snobbish about organic food or sanctimonious about processed foods. I found it amusing that she had a designer cell phone case and that when the phone rang during the appointment she answered it apologetically and had a slightly cranky conversation with one of her children. She was normal, relatable, and smart.

Jeff explained that, as people with our own food and body issues, we had avoided talking about those topics as a way of keeping them out of Bea's life. But her weight problem required management. By staying silent, we were leaving her to find her own path in the dark, which wasn't helping her at all. The doctor assured us that a child left without tools for dealing with weight gain is more likely to have disordered eating than a child to whom issues of nutrition and weight management are presented in a positive, constructive way. It's also best to help a child lose weight before puberty, when kids tend to bulk up and their body weight "set point" is established. She said the program is about giving children a foundation with which to make smart eating decisions, not making them feel bad. I was ready to sign up.

"Bea's going to be resistant to coming," I warned.

"Don't worry. I'll win her over," the nutrition doctor assured me. And I had no doubt that she would.

We made an appointment for our first consultation with the kids, and left. I was excited, and I needed Jeff to like her as much as I instantly had, and to be game to sign the family up. He did, and he was.

While I'd imagined that Jeff and I would introduce the concept of our new healthful-eating initiative to the kids together, in some sort of Norman Rockwell family moment, that's not how it panned out. With the family's inaugural appointment in January looming ever closer and my husband's evenings taken up with work, I decided to just break the news to Bea and David on my own.

I don't have any particular finesse in talking to children. I tend to speak to Bea and David like they're adults, and while I try to be loving and compassionate, my default tone is matter-of-fact and direct. Another parent might have given more thought and preparation to debuting this sensitive topic. I decided to just wing it.

It was about nine o'clock at night. The kids and I were cuddling in my bed. I went for it.

"Oh, guess what?" I said lightly. "We're going to go see someone who is going to help us eat more healthfully."

I didn't say "doctor." I didn't even say "nutritionist." But you would have thought I just announced that they both had to get kidney transplants.

"What?" Bea cried as tears sprang to her eyes. "I don't want to."

"Me neither," David chimed in, in a rare moment of agreement with his sister.

"What's the big deal?" I asked.

"We're just going because I'm fat," Bea answered.

Wow, already this was going phenomenally poorly. Should I be frank, or should I protect her feelings and maintain my flimsy ruse? What was the right thing to do? What would a good parent do?

"No, that's not it!" I insisted. "We are all going, because we all need help. Daddy eats too much at night, I want to stop drinking those stupid juices, Dave has to eat stuff other than pasta. This lady is going to teach us all how to be healthier. She's like a nutritionist."

David was bereft. "Two kids in my class went to nutritionists, and they hated it!" he complained. "They said it was like the most boring thing!" To David, something being "boring" is only slightly more acceptable than it being "extremely painful" or "potentially fatal."

"See?" I said, directing my attention to Bea and stubbornly latching on to only half of David's comment. "Lots of kids go to nutritionists! Two kids in Dave's class have gone. Daddy and I went to one once before you were even born." And, just to bolster the argument, I added: "Maddie went to one." Maddie was a skinny girl in our neighborhood whose mom had sent her to a nutritionist when she was in preschool because she only ate cheese sticks. My hope was that the more skinny kids I could come up with who went to nutritionists, the less likely it was that Bea would feel this was some sort of sentence for her being overweight.

By now they were both crying, and I felt like I had lost control of the conversation. "Guys!" I said. "It's going to be fine! We're all going to go together. It's like a New Year's resolution."

My central concern was for Bea's feelings. Until we reached the safety of the doctor's office, it was up to me to approach this topic in a positive way. Already, the kids were acting like going to this appointment was a punishment.

"Why are you crying, sweetie?" I asked Bea, caressing her cheek, ignoring David's flopping around the bed in frustration.

"I want to be able to do it myself," she whimpered.

"Do what yourself?"

"I know I need to lose weight, but I wish I could just do it myself," she said.

"I know," I said softly. "It's not your fault."

In that moment, I made the decision that I wasn't going to withhold words such as *overweight* from our discussion. I knew that word could upset her or embarrass her. But the fact that she was overweight wasn't news to her. I wanted to make sure she could see I was comfortable taking on the topic; euphemistic nomenclature smacked of unease.

I continued. "You have a health problem. You're overweight. I wish we could fix it on our own, too, but we've tried, and it didn't work. I don't know how to do it. So we're going to get someone to help us. And it's not just for you. It's for Daddy and David and me, too."

"I know it's just for me," she said.

"It's not," I insisted.

"I'm embarrassed," she whimpered.

"Look, the only reason anyone should feel embarrassed when they have an issue like this is if they don't acknowledge it," I replied. "It's brave to admit you have a problem, and smart to realize that you need someone else's help."

Silence.

"Bea, this is a problem we can fix," I told her firmly. "Lots of kids have much worse problems—diabetes or depression or cancer. Everyone has something they have to deal with, whether you realize it or not. This is your thing, and so we're going to deal with it together."

"I still don't want to go," Bea said sadly.

"Me neither!" David complained.

"Whatever, guys," I said, drained, pulling them close to me. "It's not a choice. We're going."

CHAPTER 5

I have to say that for a good minute there during the kids' outburst in response to the idea of a family nutrition reboot, I almost gave up. I thought I would just tell Jeff we needed to figure out another approach. *The kids are miserable,* I'd say. *Bea already feels singled out. This is bringing negative attention to the problem. It's becoming too big a deal.* Maybe, I thought, we should just go see the nutrition doctor in secret, and run the program on Bea surreptitiously. Maybe Jeff and I should just do the research and work we should have been doing all along about what she should eat and how much, and try feeding her that way before making a whole big dramatic issue out of it.

But I knew we had already tried our best on our own and had failed fairly spectacularly. I knew that in order to fight this disease, we needed the structure and expertise of an authority leading the way. It was the same reason I'd been successful at losing weight only when I did Weight Watchers—having guidelines to follow, going to the meetings, knowing someone else was going to be putting me on a scale and recording my weight, listening to a lecture, paying that weekly fee—those factors made all the difference for me. Even if Bea didn't need that kind of supervision, I did. And I wanted Bea to have an active role in her own treatment.

The kids' spirits lifted somewhat when they learned that for the first two appointments they'd get to leave school early. When the first meeting finally rolled around, I picked them up from school around lunchtime, and we met Jeff at the nutrition doctor's office.

The mood was grim as we sat in the waiting room. Early dismissal notwithstanding, neither Bea nor David was happy to be there. I couldn't wait for them to meet the nutrition doctor, so they could see she was cool.

She came out and greeted us, and I waited for the kids to be into her, but they were about as excited to see her as they were any other doctor, which is to say not at all. The first thing she did was weigh each of us. After I peeled off Bea's jacket and sweater, she stepped on a digital scale. I pretended to be looking at something else so as to appear nonchalant about the number, but furtively caught sight of the display, which read 93. David was under 50, and it says much about my relative concern for his weight that I can't remember the exact number, if I even bothered to look. I didn't pay any attention to what Jeff's weight was, consumed as I was with attending to the kids.

Next came the measurement of our height. Again trying to avoid the appearance of being obsessed with Bea's stats, I stole a fleeting glance at the chart, and saw the doctor write a 6 as the last number for her height. *Okay, so she's ninety-three pounds and four foot six.* I didn't remember the exact numbers from her recent pediatrician appointment, but that seemed right.

We all sat down in the consultation room. David twirled around in a leather club chair until his head was pointing downward and his feet were in the air as we answered some basic questions about what we ate and how active we were. Then it was time to see whether any of us had a metabolism issue. This part was sort of interesting to me. Bea's pediatrician had ruled out that explanation for her weight gain much earlier, but I'd always wondered whether I had a slow metabolism or a normal one, and exactly how many calories I burned in a day. A machine that resembled a laser printer with a plastic tube sticking out of it was going to tell me.

Each of us breathed into that tube for an interminable-seeming twenty minutes, then awaited the machine's output.

To the extent that we may have been hoping for a medical explanation for our family's weight struggles, we were disappointed. None of us had a metabolism problem. David's resting metabolic rate was a little faster than average. The rest of us were just normal. Later, Jeff touchingly confessed to me that he felt let down by the experiment. He'd hoped that the machine would diagnose him as having a sluggish metabolism, which would explain why he had so much trouble managing his weight.

At that point, the doctor asked Bea and David, who was by now engrossed in a game on my phone, to go into the waiting room so she could talk to Jeff and me alone.

With the kids safely out of earshot, she opened Bea's chart. "In case you were wondering," she reassured us, "you're doing the right thing by bringing her here." She divulged that Bea's BMI for age, or her body mass index plotted against that of other seven-year-olds, was in the 98th percentile. Children with a BMI for age in the 95th percentile or above are considered obese.

Obese. I found the label shocking. I almost couldn't accept it. Overweight, I could see. I was prepared for that. But this word put our family in a whole different, more alarming category. To me, obesity conjured images of 200-pound kids, limping from orthopedic complications. Was that how the medical community saw Bea?

Bea's percentile ranking was formidable, but she could hardly be considered an outlier. The statistics quantifying the extent of the childhood obesity epidemic are parroted constantly but merit repeating: at the time of this writing, one in three American children is overweight or obese. When I was a kid, 4 percent of kids ages six to eleven were obese. In 2008, 20 percent were. Chances are some of the kids you know—maybe even your own—fall into that category, whether you realize it or not.

It's easy to look at chubby kids and assume they'll grow out of their heaviness or that their size is merely an aesthetic disadvantage instead of a medical one. It feels hysterical to diagnose a child whose age is still in the single digits with a disease as dire as obesity. That may be part of why a solution to the problem is eluding us. We're unwilling to accept the severity and permanence of the disease in children so young. Especially when it falls to us to help them.

I had not previously considered the possibility that Bea was in the obese category. But in a weird way, I was strengthened by the label. It gave me a diagnosis to cling to, to excuse the inevitable deprivation that was to come. No one looks askance at the parent of a diabetic kid when she steers her child away from sugar. It can be embarrassing to see a mother grab an Almond Joy out of her kid's hand, but you can sympathize with her if you know that her son has a nut allergy. Knowing that Bea was obese officially gave her a disease that it was my responsibility to treat. What might have been construed as overzealous micromanagement could now be chalked up to good parenting. Or so I hoped and rationalized.

As we wrapped up the appointment, I purchased a copy of the

doctor's book. It had a recipe for brownies, which was one of the few desserts that had ever attracted David's interest.

"Check it out, Dave, we can make these," I said. There were also recipes for chicken Parmesan, chocolate chip cookies, and breakfast burritos. My not-so-subtle message: *This is going to be fun, kids!*

I flipped to the index of green-light values in the back of the book. The first thing I looked for was pizza. The kids regularly ate their school's pizza lunch every Friday (while I enjoyed a day off from preparing lunch), and I wanted to see how much it was going to cost them. A yellow light and a green light, apparently—whatever that meant. We had to wait until the following week to find out how many "green lights" (two of which were exchangeable for a yellow light, four of which were exchangeable for a red light) we were allotted for each meal.

But I was excited to get started with a real plan for Bea and to get my own weight back down to the level I'd grown accustomed to. I felt a kind of adrenaline-fueled exhilaration. This was familiar territory for me: the first few days of a new diet, full of hope and anticipation, where the food shopping felt fun, and even words such as *tablespoon* in the recipes for the new diet foods sounded tasty. Best of all, I wasn't doing it on my own—I had teammates!

We walked out of the office into the midday sunshine.

"Should we get lunch?" Jeff asked. The question chilled me. Well, yes, of course we should get lunch. But what would be an appropriate lunch for our situation? What was "lunch" going to mean from now on? We were about to spend a week in this weird limbo, knowing we were eating too much and not yet knowing how much less we should eat.

As we always do when we want to eat light, we decided to get Japanese food. We found ourselves at a table at a busy, dark, ramen restaurant. As Jeff and the kids looked at their menus, I paged through the food index of the book I'd just purchased, to look up the traffic-light values of various Japanese dishes.

"Edamame is free!" I exclaimed. "We can have as much of it as we want."

"Cool!" Jeff chimed in, while the kids ignored us.

We ordered edamame. And soup, and shrimp tempura, and sushi, and chicken teriyaki. I added up the green lights, not knowing what the target was, but knowing we were undoubtedly exceeding it. But I was unprepared to justify a change in our usual ordering habits just yet.

It was strange that first week, holding the keys to the program in our hands but not actually knowing how much we were allowed to eat. It was like having a vial of pills for our disease but not knowing the dosage. Bea wouldn't talk much about it, but David was oddly into it. One day at home, he spent half an hour making a pen-and-ink drawing of the cover of our new nutrition bible, inscribing it with the motivational phrase "Let's eat healthy!"

At some point David and Bea asked me what their BMIs were, and together we located them on a chart in the book. Days later, upon opening the book to find a recipe, I noticed two slivers of yellow Post-it notes that David had carefully attached to the relevant pages. *Dave is healthy weight,* the first one read, written in David's small, tidy handwriting and affixed to the boys' BMI chart. The other, pasted alongside the girls' chart in the same handwriting, read simply, "Bea is obese."

So Bea knew she was not just overweight but obese. She also knew that this "nutritional regimen" she was on is what grownups commonly called a "diet." I had the same attitude toward these words as I did toward telling Bea she was, indeed, "overweight." Once it became clear that Bea's problem wasn't going to be addressed by changes barely discernible to her, such as extra activity and more fruits and vegetables, it didn't make sense to shy away from frank terminology in discussing the issue.

This fear of calling a spade a spade reminded me of when Bea and David were in preschool and had to take a couple of standardized tests that are required of children in New York City seeking admission to selective public schools. The conventional wisdom was, *For God's sake, don't let your child know he's taking a test! Tell him he's going to do "special work with a teacher," or meeting with "a lady who is interested in finding out what four-year-olds know." But not a test!*

That's what I don't get. Since when is my four-year-old aware of what "test" means? And to the extent that he is, is the association necessarily negative? What "tests" has he really been exposed to at this point? A hearing test? A test of his reflexes? I hardly think the word is conjuring an image of sitting in a lecture hall with a blue test booklet in front of him, sweating over organic chemistry problems. So why can't we just call it a test and present the word as a neutral thing—maybe even a good thing?

When my kids found out in kindergarten that they were getting "homework," they were elated! Couldn't wait. It was something big kids got to do. It was cool to them. Words that have negative connotations to us do not necessarily have those same associations for our children. I really didn't understand why people seemed to think their kids were going to freak out and blow their kindergarten assessments if they thought of it as a "test."

Growing up, I remember being annoyed at the value judgment inherent in descriptive terms about someone's physique. Why aren't "fat" and "thin" as neutrally applied as "tall" and "short"? Why is what is socially considered to be "normal" such a narrow sliver of what is medically accepted to be normal? I should be able to describe people as "fat" if they are, indeed, fat, without that being considered an insult. Similarly, if I call people "thin," they should be assumed to be as deviant from the norm as the people I just called "fat." And individuals who are "normal"—which is a wider swath of people than most of society will acknowledge—are neither thin nor fat.

Meanwhile, shouldn't "diet" connote what it literally means: the kind of food that a person normally eats every day? Like a vegetarian diet or a gluten-free diet. Why is it automatically assumed to refer to a weight-loss effort? I wanted to take the charge out of these words so that they weren't so painful to hear.

Another example of how I felt our culture has fallen off the rails a bit with regard to these issues: I can't even begin to zip up my mother's size-8 dresses from the 1960s, but now if I go to the Gap, I'm sometimes a size small. If I'm a small, what are the loads of women who are way, way thinner than I am wearing? (The answer, apparently, can be found in the existence of inane new sizes including XXS and 00.) I assume that size numbering has evolved to protect women's egos as we've gotten heavier as a population, but is that a good thing? We're also served larger sodas and bigger portions of food than we used to be, because we like to eat more. Whole industries have changed to accommodate our new level of unhealthiness, instead of pushing to alleviate it.

People often tell me I look "thin," and it's impossible to tell whether that's some sort of complimentary way of saying "average weight" or whether they truly think I am below normal. Then, of course, we're supposed to feel great when someone calls us "skinny," a word that really should have a negative connotation. And some women actually take it as a compliment when, after dropping a few pounds, someone remarks that they look "anorexic."

I feel bad using the word *fat* around overweight people (see, I was just too scared to call them fat, and I'm only speaking hypothetically!), and it's a reflection on everyone's discomfort with acknowledging weight issues. If a fat person says, like so many of us do, "I'm fat," there's this impulse to rush to contradict her. "No, you're not!" we want to say, because somehow the word itself is so cutting. But is "You're not fat!" the correct response when the person is, indeed, objectively fat?

In our discussions of this issue, Bea and I usually used the word *overweight*, which seemed to strike the appropriate balance between colloquial and medical. It was less harsh-sounding than *fat* and less clinical than *obese*. But Bea knew where she fell on the BMI chart, and while I assured her we were going to get her to a healthy weight, the knowledge that she was different, that she had this problem with a weird name, was hard for her to take.

One evening we were chatting about her day at school when she got quiet, then teary. I asked what she was thinking about that was making her sad.

"We were all reading this magazine at school and it was talking about how unhealthy school lunches were," she explained. "And there's a section in all the articles that tells you some tricky words. And one of the words was *obese*. And after we read the thing, my teacher said, 'None of you in this class are obese.' And it just made me really sad because I know that I am, and I'm just trying to change that. And it's so hard. I just want to blend in with everyone."

At moments like this, I faltered in my confidence about my approach. I knew she was sad because she felt different. But were her tears from the feeling of being overweight or from the struggle of fighting against it? Was she crying because she was obese or because I had forced her to acknowledge her disease and how difficult it was to change? Was the work we were doing together bringing her to tears or helping to get her to a point where there wasn't anything to cry about? I wasn't sure.

Ultimately, I knew that we had to keep trying to get to a place where she was physically healthy and emotionally happy. The nutrition doctor's office seemed the right starting point. When we returned there the next week, we were seen by an associate nutritionist, an upbeat, professional young woman. Bea and I were each a few ounces lighter, thanks to the stabs in the dark I had made at reducing our food intake. David and Jeff weighed in, too, but I couldn't tell you what the scale said because again, really, I was only concerned with Bea's status.

I do, however, remember what Bea was wearing when she stepped on the scale: a T-shirt and leggings. This was important because I knew that, from that moment on, I was going to have to make sure she dressed in a similar outfit every Friday to eliminate the chance that the variable of her clothing would affect the results of her weigh-in.

During my five months on Weight Watchers after David was born, I made sure that I wore a short-sleeved T-shirt and jersey drawstring pants to every weekly meeting, regardless of the weather. As a seasoned self-weigher, I had a pretty good idea of how many pounds an outfit could add. My beloved Weight Watchers meeting leader used to joke that when she was trying to lose weight, she'd even hesitate before putting on lipstick prior to stepping on the scale. And while I wasn't quite going that far, I was not about to let a wool turtleneck or a pair of thick socks stand in the way of an accurate weight reading for any of us.

The problem was that our appointments were going to be after school. My preference would have been to weigh in at the beginning of the day, before eating or drinking anything. Tracking our weight at 4:00 p.m. every Friday seemed to provide many opportunities for misleading results. What if Bea had a big snack on her way to the appointment, or even just drank a bottle of water, and it showed up on the scale? What if someone had celebrated a birthday at school and her weight reflected a fluke cupcake? These issues concerned me, but there was no way around them.

After we were weighed, I eagerly took possession of the pages listing how many green lights we got at each meal. Bea's chart and mine were almost identical. We got two green lights for breakfast, three for lunch, and one for each of two snacks. While Bea got three green lights at dinner, I got four. David got several more green lights, since he wasn't trying to lose weight. And because of his size relative to the rest of us, Jeff got the most green lights of all, including a whopping seven at dinner.

Despite our divergent heights, weights, and ages, Bea and I were not so different metabolically. The calorimetry test had revealed her resting metabolic rate burned about 1,500 calories per day, and I burned about 1,700. By my calculations, the charts the nutritionist handed to us converted to about 1,400 calories a day for Bea and 1,600 calories a day for me, if you account for both the allotted green lights and the calories one could expect to take in under the program's fruit and vegetables policy, which required some be eaten at each meal and snack, and allowed unlimited consumption at other times of day. So if you subtract that from our daily caloric burn, the plan called for us to take in about 100 calories fewer each day than we were expending.

Based on the formula that 3,500 calories equals a pound, at that pace, we'd lose about a pound a month, which is a moderate rate of weight loss for kids and a depressingly slow rate for me. The nutritionist assured us we could bump the rate of weight loss up to a half pound a week if we increased our activity level. Healthy, but still slow.

I asked about the unlimited fruit, knowing how my family could put away bananas and oranges. The associate nutritionist assured us it was very unusual for anyone on the program to consume so much fruit that it would impede weight loss. Jeff assured her he could easily do so. She said we should see how it went, and we could adjust if we found it was becoming a problem.

Back at home, Bea and I flipped through the nutrition doctor's book, seeking inspiration among the recipes. I headed to the supermarket and stocked up on diet-friendly foods. I bought pounds and pounds of fruit: oranges, apples, bananas, strawberries, grapes, melon. I filled the refrigerator with carrots, lettuce, tomatoes, and cucumbers. I chopped up vegetables and cooked them in broth to make a "free" soup. It was time-consuming. And pricey.

I learned, for the first time in my life, what kinds of apples I liked and didn't like. I'd eaten them infrequently and certainly never bought them, so it was interesting to learn that they offered so much variation. The green ones were too tart for me, but Bea loved them. I preferred the sweet Galas. Honeycrisps were David's favorites, but they were hard to find where we live. Who knew that comparing apples to apples was so complicated?

In response to some consumers' desire for portion control, snack manufacturers have begun meting out their cookies, chips, and crackers into individually packaged 100-calorie snack packs. Pleasantly surprised to see that any one of them was a green light, suitable for Bea's allocated morning or after-school snacks, I began to rethink my lockstep disdain for foods that come in sealed bags within cardboard boxes. In a world where Bea was going to have to hear the word *no* a lot, it dawned on me that these little doctor-sanctioned doses of nutritional vice could help keep her from feeling deprived. I threw aside my ingrained cultural shame about feeding kids processed foods and bought a wide array: fudge-stripe cookies, chocolate-covered pretzels, Doritos, Cheez-It crackers, Honey Maid cinnamon thin crisps. Packaged foods I would have been ashamed to be seen buying previously now held a certain uneasy place in my heart, and in Bea's diet.

Here is how our daily meals started to evolve:

BREAKFAST

We all had two green lights to spend, and Bea and I generally invested them in high-fiber cereal and skim milk, a mini bagel with low-fat cream cheese, or, when we had time to actually cook something, oatmeal or an egg and whole-wheat toast. David continued to eat his preferred bagel and cream cheese, cereal and skim milk, or baguette slices with light butter. He insisted on being served a larger portion, which I acceded to since he always left some of it over, with the result that he ate the same amount we did. Jeff made himself eggs and toast.

MORNING SNACK

Bea and I would have a 100-calorie pack and a piece of fruit, she at school and me at home. David didn't have a snack period at school, so I applied his green light to his after-school snack.

LUNCH

An ever-evolving project, lunch for Bea tended to contain one serving of protein (salami, turkey bacon, chicken), reduced-calorie bread or a small tortilla, a piece of fruit, some raw vegetables, and some little "extra," be it a wedge of low-fat cheese or a few crackers.

David ate five pigs in blankets, an orange, cooked carrots, pretzels or breadsticks, and a 90-calorie Rice Krispies Treat. Every day. He's a creature of habit.

I would eat a toasted light English muffin with melted nonfat cheese and a poached egg, with a slice of tomato and onion. Or a Smuckers Uncrustables peanut butter and jelly sandwich. Or a six-piece tuna sushi roll with no avocado, since the avocado jacked up the meal another traffic light.

Given that he was eating on the go at work, some days Jeff had a salad for lunch, and other days he ate a large restaurant meal. He claimed that either this diet would work for him or it wouldn't, but given that we ate so many meals apart, he felt it was impractical for me to manage his choices too much.

AFTERNOON SNACK

David usually had a slice of pizza or a frozen fruit bar. For Bea, I innovated green-light s'mores, using two chocolate graham crackers, a marshmallow, and our toaster-oven broiler. They were delicious and she ate them almost every day. Plus fruit.

DINNER

Dinner was a challenge. More so than ever before, I became a short-order cook to suit everyone's needs. I needed to make two full and separate meals every night. I would carefully research and craft a diet-friendly entrée for Bea, her father, and me, then throw together a pasta-based dish with some protein and vegetables for David. David might dine on meatballs and spaghetti, chicken cutlets with broccoli, or pasta and Brussels sprouts. The rest of us would enjoy something like chicken tikka masala, turkey meatloaf, or Korean barbecue beef in lettuce wraps.

I know it was a failure of my parenting not to work harder to force David to eat what everyone else was eating, but my duty was to provide all members of the family with a meal they liked that met their nutritional needs. Getting David to accept a wider variety of foods was a nice goal, but there's no way around the reality that it took a definite backseat to the more urgent requirement of helping Bea get healthy.

I was exhausted by the arguments over food that came at me from all sides, so I tried to preempt at least some of them by not serving David anything that was "too spicy" (read: contained any seasoning other than salt) or in some other way didn't meet the narrow preferences of his palate. It was easier to cook a second dinner. And he always ate a healthful, well-balanced meal. It was just usually a different one than the rest of us had. I told myself that once Bea's eating was squared away, my focus could and would shift to addressing David's pickiness.

I'm no great chef, but I did sort of enjoy finding recipes that Bea and her dad would like and that could be served in a reasonable portion size but still come in under 300 calories. As if food wasn't taking up enough of my attention when I was at home, it was also the focus of my work hours, as I reviewed that unedited cooking show footage. I was often so taken with the recipe being prepared on-screen that I'd be inspired to make it myself. And I noticed that while the chefs would sometimes talk about how healthful the dishes were, they were never specifically trying to make them low-calorie. So I started doing it myself—scaling down portion sizes and substituting ingredients so that these meals would be appropriate for a family with an overweight child.

We tried some new recipes, with varying levels of success. Some things did not benefit much calorically from being made "healthful," and the trade-off in taste was not worthwhile. The much-anticipated brownie recipe from the nutrition doctor's book was a huge disappointment. It required pitted dates, which not only were nearly impossible to find but also gave the finished product the disturbing mouth-feel of what I imagine it must be like to eat roaches. So what if they were only one green light each? So were two Entenmann's Little Bites brownies, which are far more yummy, or a small homemade brownie baked with the old dieter's substitute of unsweetened applesauce for the oil. So why bother with the pitted dates?

I also didn't see the benefit of making chicken nuggets breaded in instant mashed potato flakes, as the nutrition doctor's recipe dictated, rather than, say, panko or bread crumbs. But some new things we tried were winners. The black bean burger was a revelation, with complex flavor from cumin and cilantro and a satisfying chew. The turkey sloppy Joes I adapted from an online recipe, inspired by something in the doctor's book, became a staple that I cooked nearly every week.

Most of Bea's dinners were about half the size of what they had been. And a difficult question came up that first official week on the program—one that would recur more times during the coming months. As I placed food in front of the children at any meal, Bea would regard the contents of her plate and compare it with David's, instantly realizing he was getting twice what she was.

"That's not fair!" she cried. "Why does Dave get [insert inequitable food distribution allegation here]?" He would get two pieces of chicken and she would get only one. David would have a full-size bagel, while Bea got a mini. He'd have pasta, she'd have only vegetables.

The obvious truth was, of course, that she needed to lose weight and he didn't. They both knew that. And connecting food intake with weight gain and loss is a reasonable life lesson. If you want to lose weight, you have to eat less. But when you're hungry and you love food and your brother's plate has twice as much food on it as yours does, that answer isn't entirely satisfactory. It explains the reasoning but doesn't address the unfairness.

Sometimes I'd hide behind science and say, "Because you have different nutritional needs." Sometimes I'd try to make it sound like she didn't really get less food: "Dave only eats half of what we give him, so you end up eating the same amount." And sometimes I'd pass the buck and say, "Because the doctor says you can eat that much, but David gets a little more." I was happy to have someone to put the blame on, since otherwise I was usually absorbing all the resentment.

Whatever I said, though, Bea was right. It wasn't fair.

I relocated my extra dinner green light to earlier in the day so that my plate looked identical to Bea's. And my husband received double what we did. That way, I could ally myself with Bea and share in the unfairness she felt. The same way she looked at her brother's plate, I could point to Jeff's plate.

"I wish I could eat what Daddy does, but I can't," I commiserated.

"If you eat like me, you're going to look like me," her dad teased.

"I'm eating the same amount you are," I told her. "I know it's not a lot. But it's enough. Eat it and see if you're actually still hungry."

She always was. Whereas my body was used to small portions and I could be satisfied after a tiny slider burger or a bowl of soup,

Bea's body still had to adjust. It wasn't an easy transition, and I heard about it plenty.

I also went a bit overboard at first, trying to make the program appealing by translating as many green lights as possible into junky, kid-friendly food. That first week, we never exceeded our green-light quota, but processed snacks accounted for three or four of Bea's ten green lights per day.

I quickly realized this was my own pathology projected onto her. Bea has a far more varied palate than I do. Sugary snacks, while welcome, are not necessarily superior in her estimation to, say, hummus and carrots. I tried to remind myself of this as I planned out her meals. She didn't always share my proclivity for indulgence over quantity, and it was incumbent upon me to instill good habits in her. But I would kick myself anytime she asked for a dessert after dinner and I had squandered a green light on some stupid salad dressing that I could have saved for a Skinny Cow ice cream bar.

I was pleased with how that first week went. There were no major meltdowns, no seismic shifts in how our household operated. All of us had eaten foods we liked, in quantities that generally satisfied us. Bea had been a champ at adhering to the program, eating what I gave her and grudgingly accepting my limit setting when she asked for more.

The kids and I headed in to see the nutrition doctor after that week. This was the first time they hadn't had the privilege of missing school for the appointment. They were irked that this nutrition thing was impinging on the first hours of their weekend.

Are you coming to meet us? I texted Jeff when he was a no-show in the waiting room. No response.

I had brought Bea a small snack bar to eat en route to the

appointment—something with little weight, so it wouldn't show up on the scale. I couldn't bring myself to look as she weighed in.

"Lost almost a pound!" the doctor announced.

It wasn't a huge amount of weight. And secretly I'd been hoping for a full pound loss. But it was a decisive move in the right direction and certainly a faster loss than the projected one or two pounds a *month*. I felt relieved. The machine had been set in motion.

As our consultation with the doctor ended, my phone beeped with a text from Jeff: *Just got out of a meeting. Sorry. Can I join you now?*

Never mind, I typed. *We're finished.*

As we left the office, I knew that the level of enthusiasm and privacy we'd enjoyed during the first week on the program could not last. We weren't always going to feel so motivated, and I wasn't always going to be able to control every meal. Things were going to get harder.

CHAPTER 6

One night the whole family went to our friends' house for dinner, joining a number of other couples and a large contingent of kids.

The kids ate first: pasta and vegetables. I carefully portioned out an acceptably small dish of penne with Parmesan and sparingly served Bea some vegetables, which had been prepared with oil and therefore were not the "free" vegetables we ate at home. While David ate a large portion—penne with Parmesan being one of his all-time favorites—Bea's dinner was pretty tiny, because unlike David, she wanted to have dessert, too. Which she did, before running off to play with the other kids.

We adults hung out in the kitchen as my good friend prepared our dinner, Niçoise salad. She peeled and sliced hard-boiled eggs, spooned glistening tuna onto salad greens, added tender chunks of boiled potatoes, threw in some olives, and dressed it all with some great olive oil. It looked absolutely delicious.

With Bea safely out of earshot, I told the assembled friends about our new food strategy and how Bea was understandably grouchy about it. I pointed out how she had complained about how much smaller her pasta serving was than anyone else's, and how it was hard for her and tough for us to see her go through that frustration, but that it seemed necessary. Our friends were uniformly sympathetic and supportive. They all made Jeff and me feel like we were doing the right thing.

We sat down to eat. The salad was amazing.

A few minutes later Bea came into the room.

"I'm hungry," she said.

I didn't know what kind of fruits or vegetables our friends might have on hand, and I didn't want to bother them with having to serve her any. Frankly, I didn't want to bother myself with having to serve her any. She had just had dinner. And dessert. The adults had just started eating.

Bea's request for food also seemed to take on a searing significance in the wake of what I'd just shared with the grown-ups. I suddenly felt like there was a spotlight shining on us. I imagined that while everyone was continuing to eat, they were also intently listening to see how I would react to this tricky situation.

"You had dinner already," I reminded her.

"But I'm hungry," Bea said. It was a routine we'd gone through many times, but never in front of other people.

"Do you want some salad?" the hostess asked readily.

"No, thanks," I interrupted quickly. "She already ate dinner."

"I'm still hungry," Bea pointed out.

"Maybe you could have like a piece of fruit . . . ," I said, my eyes scanning the kitchen.

"If she's hungry, she can have some salad," my friend offered again.

"Okay," said Bea.

I stared at the salad. I hadn't yet calculated the traffic light content of the small bowl I had served myself. I figured that the tuna was a green light or a yellow light. The potatoes and eggs, another green. The olive oil, a green or yellow. Then there were the olives, and how many olives equaled a green light again?

"I'm sorry. Bea," I interjected. "It's got a lot of dressing on it, and—"

"Just olive oil!" my friend interrupted. "It's super healthy!"

I forced a grim smile. "I know, but—"

"Just a little!" my friend insisted, and pushed the bowl into Bea's eager hands.

I didn't know what to do. My friend was being a hospitable dinner hostess, responding caringly to a child complaining of being hungry. I was trying to be a good mother, an advocate for my child's health. But I also wanted to be a polite dinner guest. Bea happily devoured the salad as I sat silently.

Long afterward, my friend who'd hosted us that night and I discussed this incident. I described it as one of the many ways our food issues turned social situations stressful as I tried to navigate the triangle between what other people thought I should feed Bea, what I thought was best for her, and what Bea wanted to eat.

"I can't believe how pushy I was!" my friend marveled in retrospect.

"You only did what any normal person would do in that situation," I assured her.

Overseeing the diet of an overweight child is an uneasy position to be in. It is going to cause social strain. I readily admit that I am not the most socially adept person, and I don't handle tension well. While I felt I had failed Bea that night by eventually capitulating to the Niçoise salad, there was certainly no blame to be placed on anyone else.

But I was mad at myself for not being more protective. I felt bad that I'd let her eat food we hadn't planned on, just to avoid some social discomfort. It wasn't the one bowl of salad that worried me. It was the very real fear that not sticking to our strategy 100 percent, all the time, left the door open for more such moments to creep in. I'd been on enough diets myself and had tried enough halfhearted measures with Bea to realize what was required. The salad incident served as a reminder that if we took our commitment to the rules of our program too lightly, the entire endeavor would collapse. I had to think like an alcoholic trying to stay on the wagon. One drink is too many, and a thousand is not enough.

So the next time, I spoke up. We were at Bea's cousin's birthday party. I saw her heading for the M&M bowl on the buffet table, even before lunch was served.

"Hey!" I shouted. And, though grinning, I widened my eyes and opened up my hands as if to say, *What the hell?* Bea caught my gaze, coyly slipped a few of the M&Ms into her mouth, and ran off.

When the kids sat down to lunch, each place setting featured a juice box. I replaced Bea's with a water bottle.

"Aww, I want the juice!" she whined.

"I know, but it's just *juice,*" I said with an exaggerated sneer, sending up its inconsequence, trying to forge an intimate camaraderie over the idea of wasting calories on a drink—like all the other kids were ignorant for mindlessly drinking what they were given, whereas she was the clever strategist. "We're going to have cake soon! So let's just drink water." She didn't argue. I knew she wasn't really into juice anyway, so that was an easy savings.

When the cake was served, Bea literally licked her plate clean. David turned his piece over to me after a few bites.

"I don't like it," he said, as if it had been a dose of cough medicine.

"No?" I asked innocently, taking a bite as though doing so for verification purposes. I ate the entire rest of the piece just to be sure it wasn't bad.

Amid the frantic goodbyes, goody-bag distribution, jacket-locating, happy birthday wishes, and general post-sugar-consumption mayhem, I saw Bea approach the buffet table again. She was staring at the cookie plate. I pushed my way through the crowd, calling out to her.

"Bea! What are you doing?" I said, raising my voice above the din.

"I want a cookie," she said simply.

"You can't have a cookie," I said.

"Why not?" she asked. She knew why not.

"You just had cake! We had a whole discussion about what you were going to eat here. You could have had the cookies, the cake, or the M&Ms, but you cannot have all of them. You picked the cake. You're done."

I'm not sure anyone actually paid attention to us. But I understood that if they had, they might have found the exchange embarrassing. The high-strung mom nagging her overweight daughter about cookies and candy. I imagined their thoughts:

Jesus, lady, what is your problem? Just let her have the stupid cookies. She's seven years old. This is her childhood. Childhood is cookies and birthday cake. Eating cookies is not a disease; it's a small and simple pleasure. You are ruining her innocent years by making every treat a sin. Did you ever weigh the damage of your nagging eye against her buoyancy and joy?

God, yes. I considered that point of view every day. There were countless moments of refusing, denying, questioning, and bargaining between Bea and me. Instances when she was asked to take responsibility for controlling her eating when other kids were reveling in the pleasure of not having to think about it. I persisted despite incessant doubts because, I told myself, the end result would be worthwhile, and that in its way, my pestering her was not just annoying, it was important.

To me, intervening when I saw Bea about to make a bad choice needed to become a reflexive reaction, like seeing her about to wander into a busy street. I didn't know if this anti-obesity undertaking could really work, but I did know that it was sure to fail if I gave in "just this once." Being the killjoy around food was not fun, and it wasn't how I was naturally inclined to act. But it was a crucial part of the process for Bea. In order to keep her resolve strong, my will could not bend.

It called to mind when my kids were toddlers and I went to all those workshops their preschools offered on parenting. You know how it is when you're a new parent: you read the books, scan the online message boards, and attend the lectures in hopes that someone will tell you how to raise your kids right.

The first workshop I attended was on sleep training. As with almost every other behavioral issue with children, including potty training, limit setting, and sibling relations, the parenting expert exhorted us to be consistent. If the child toddles out of her room when she's supposed to be going to sleep, you wordlessly bring her back to bed. Make the mistake of smiling and greeting her and letting her play for a few minutes, and your authority is shot. Let her cuddle in your bed for one night, and you're back to square one, having lost all credibility as a disciplinarian. Kids need to know what the limits are and that their parents will enforce them. It's actually scary for a child, the expert told us, to feel there are no parameters. They are not equipped to run your household, she said. So don't let them.

When I make a deal with one of my kids, I expect that child to hold up his or her end of the bargain. If they promise to take their baths once they complete a round of Othello, I am not pleased if I walk in ten minutes later and find they've finished the game and started a new one. If a trip to the movies is contingent upon their not getting into a fight all morning, the outing is canceled the moment one kid provokes a sibling argument. Homework is done before computer games are played, period.

Every day our family engages in multiple tiny negotiations, and I take some pride in delivering on my promises and following through on my threats. Though sleep training may have been the exception to the rule (you'll recall the ten or eleven o'clock bedtimes mentioned earlier), I didn't just sit through those toddler-parenting workshops—I took them to heart. If I commit to something, my consistency is pretty consistent.

If all of Bea's meals had been prepared and served by me and eaten in private, our weight-loss journey would have been a radically different experience. But food is public. Food is social. Ultimately I was going to have to let Bea eat with, and under the supervision of, other people. The prospect caused me some anxiety. I didn't trust anyone else to understand her dietary requirements, let alone love her enough to protect her progress. So I didn't let go of the apron strings easily.

But while these minor public scuffles over food weren't fun, I don't think they were so different from the mom-versus-kid limit-setting disagreements many other families engaged in over sweets. What did get significantly more stressful were the times when I had turned Bea over to the care of another adult and returned to find that bad choices had been made while she wasn't on my watch.

At those times I felt frustrated and helpless that I couldn't control everything.

Part of the problem was that communicating Bea's nutritional needs to others was a delicate matter. At first I was up front about it. I clearly and forthrightly told whatever grown-up I was leaving in charge what the situation was, as though it were no big deal.

"What were you guys going to do for a snack?" I asked her best friend's mom as Bea and her little pal prepared to go off on a playdate together one afternoon.

"I don't know," the friend's mom answered. I should mention Bea's best friend is a skinny kid.

"Okay, because Bea should pretty much just have fruit or some vegetables. Maybe a small snack, like under a hundred calories," I said.

"How about a yogurt?" the mom suggested.

"Ehhh . . . ," I said, grimacing. Yogurt was one of those foods whose diet value was, in my opinion, overrated. A regular container of low-fat yogurt is a yellow light on our program—and Bea only gets one green light for snack. If she ate a 4-ounce container of fat-free yogurt, she could get it down to a green light. "A small one," I allowed.

"Okay," the mom said as Bea rolled her eyes at the indignity of the conversation.

"If you had a peanut allergy, I would be telling your friends' parents that you couldn't have anything with nuts," I insisted later, when we discussed it one-on-one. "Your problem is that you are overweight, so you can't have things with lots of calories. It's not that different."

Iron-clad logic, right? Bea didn't see it my way. She thought I was being annoying, unfair, and a drag.

I understood her feelings, and I see how obesity *is* annoying, unfair, and a drag. But guess what? Life isn't fair. Imparting that wisdom to our children is an inevitable part of parenting. Obesity is a medical condition, not just an aesthetic one. It can be a life-threatening disease, so it makes sense that we would treat it as such. No one should be any more embarrassed by it than they are to have epilepsy or ADHD. Was the declaration of being on a diet an admission of being overweight? Was admitting being overweight any more humiliating (or obvious) than just *being* overweight? Wasn't it less embarrassing to acknowledge it and let people know you were aware of the problem and doing something about it?

My MO has always been two-pronged: cover up my flaws as best I can, then lay them out on the table for discussion to expose my insecurity preemptively. Throughout all the years that I've battled with my weight, even as I sought to hide my body under layers of obfuscating clothing, I fessed up about my feelings to others. I was the girl you could overhear groaning, "Ugh, I am *so fat*," as I patted my distended belly. In the same way, if I had an obvious pimple on my face, I would attack it with concealer, then find a way to work it into conversation, just so everyone knew that I knew that they noticed it, and they shouldn't feel awkward about it.

I'm not saying this is the best way to disarm people's judgment, but it was *my* coping mechanism. And there was something of a vigilante feeling about it. I was acknowledging the existence of potbellied, pimply people and identifying as one of them. I wasn't going so far as to be out and *proud*, but at least I was out.

In Bea's case, to allay the potential awkwardness involved in discussing an obese child's dietary restrictions, I wanted to be very plainspoken about our predicament. But Bea wasn't a fan of that approach, so I usually confined my dictates about what Bea could eat to phone calls, text messages, or emails with her friends' parents or caregivers before the playdate started. The problem, however, was that even when the information was communicated, parents of kids who were not overweight often failed to grasp the gist or strictness of Bea's eating limitations.

The most common mistake was that the grown-up in charge would think, *Okay, I got it, Bea needs to eat healthful snacks.* Which all too often ended up in the land of 300-calorie snacks of yogurt and almonds. Almonds, like yogurt, have enjoyed some kick-ass PR over the past few years, emerging as an ideal, all-natural combination of fiber, protein, and good fats in a handy, portable size. The only problem is that at seven calories per tiny nut, a handful of them can easily reach 200 calories. A yellow light. Double what Bea is allowed for a snack. And it's basically like bird food. So unless you're really into almonds, I don't know why you'd want to eat them as a snack if you're a kid trying to lose weight. But nuts found their way into Bea's hands on a few playdates.

Other parents took my request for a "small" snack to heart, but missed the mark. A "little" ice cream cone—which a mom fully aware of our weight-loss effort once bought for Bea—doesn't quite cut it. Indeed, what passes for a small snack to most parents—frozen yogurt, an individual-size bag of Pirate's Booty, cheese and crackers—seems totally legitimate until you break down the calorie content and see it's two or three times what Bea is allowed.

I understood then and I understand all the more now that no one other than someone deeply involved in this kind of effort can easily grasp the specifics: how few calories an overweight child is allowed when she's trying to lose weight, how controlled portion sizes need to be for a child who is inclined to overeat. Bea's allotted calories could be squandered and exceeded so easily. I knew that if everyone who provided Bea with food let just a few extra bites slide, that would add up to a whole lot of excess food over time.

I know, generally, that parents and babysitters genuinely thought they were giving Bea something that was healthful and diet friendly. Certainly they shouldn't have to deprive their own children of ice cream, almonds, or anything else they're used to, just because they've been nice enough to invite Bea over. But for me, as a parent trying to manage every snack, it's an understatement to say it's a challenge.

For Bea, who was there to play and who would no doubt much rather join in fully while there, all this could be confusing and burdensome. What was she supposed to do when presented with a snack she coveted, which her friend was eating, and which a grown-up entrusted with her care had chosen for her? Of course she accepted the snack every time. And then I would show up, and a little hell would break loose.

One day I came to pick Bea up from gymnastics class. She'd gone there with her friend and her friend's babysitter, who'd provided the girls with a snack en route. I'd texted the babysitter earlier in the day and asked her to limit Bea's snack to 100 calories, plus any fresh fruits and vegetables. She'd confirmed that was what she'd do.

When I showed up, I watched the last few minutes of class. After having found a succession of leotards too uncomfortable at the beginning of the semester, Bea had opted to wear a T-shirt and leggings to every class. As she stretched and jumped alongside a dozen normal-to-underweight girls in sleek gymnastics outfits, their images reflected in the mirror that spanned the wall of the studio, I wondered if she felt different. Was her decision to forgo a leotard truly a comfort-driven decision, or was there some element of wanting to hide her body?

My heart swelled as I watched her gamely execute her calisthenics, occasionally tripping over her feet but recovering with a big smile. As class ended, she ran over to me, and I enveloped her in a proud hug. As I helped her put on her shoes, she resumed eating the snack she'd apparently started before class: a cup of ramen noodle soup.

I know it seems like a total overreaction, but at the time I was so thrown by the sight of this cup of noodles that I almost couldn't focus my eyes on Bea's shoes.

"Where did you get that?" I asked.

"It was my snack," Bea said, pausing from her slurping.

"You cannot eat that," I said, quietly but sharply. "Why are you eating that?"

"Okay, okay," she said, putting down the noodles. We stood up to leave, and I mumbled a distracted thank-you and goodbye to Bea's friend and her babysitter.

"Sorry," Bea said as we walked down the hallway lobby.

And then I felt totally stupid. It wasn't Bea's fault she had eaten some noodles her friend's babysitter had given her. It wasn't the babysitter's fault that she had incorrectly surmised it was a reasonable snack. Maybe it was my fault for not having sent Bea to class with something to eat. Maybe it wasn't anybody's fault.

Moments before, the fact that Bea had sucked down a 300-calorie soup seemed to upend everything we'd been working for. But Bea's sweet, totally unnecessary apology made me realize I couldn't make her feel bad about it.

"I shouldn't have gotten so upset," I said. "You didn't do anything wrong. I'm sorry."

We walked past a table where a couple of young students were hosting a bake sale to raise money for their gymnastics team.

"Oh," Bea said, gesturing to the baked goods for sale. "I also had a cookie. I had a dollar in my backpack. And I asked the girls, 'What on this table costs a dollar?' and they said, '*Everything* is a dollar!' So I got a cookie."

It makes me laugh when I think about it now, but at that moment it sure didn't seem funny. I felt defeated. The cookie bumped her snack up to a red light. She'd exceeded her snack allowance by the same amount of food she was allotted for dinner.

I didn't make her feel bad about the cookie, but I had to account for it somehow. I felt the day starting to crumble nutritionally, and with it, the week. It was like when I was in high school and worried about blowing an exam. I rationalized my panic: that one test would affect my grade that quarter, which would affect my annual report card, which would affect my grade point average, which would affect my chances of getting into the college of my choice, which might affect my future career. These mistakes had a way of snowballing in my mind. I had to figure out how to correct our course.

So back at home, after a brief hesitation, I scraped the pasta off her dinner plate, leaving her only a small piece of chicken and vegetables to eat. I didn't do it as a punishment—I believed she ate those noodles innocently (the cookie was another story, but I let that count as her afternoon snack). I had to be the tough one and enforce the rules. Ramen and cookie for snack equals no pasta with dinner. It was an important accounting, not just for her as the eater of the food but also for me as the server of the food.

I vowed to make an effort to be understanding about her occasional errors in judgment. I had to remember she was a kid and that I was asking for adult-size levels of maturity and responsibility from her. But I did feel it was important to teach her that she can't go through life expecting grown-ups to make all her food decisions for her. She needed to take all she had learned about herself and food over these months and say no when it's appropriate, or be willing to trade out something else later.

But tension could arise even when I was the one making the food choices. Because, quite simply, our family's decision to make Cool Whip Free and Diet Coke part of our children's diets rubbed some other parents the wrong way.

CHAPTER 7

During one of my early reconnaissance missions to the supermarket, I discovered sugar-free whipped cream, which, at only five calories for two tablespoons, seemed like a minor miracle. It turned our boring bowls of strawberries into towering parfaits for a scant ten or twenty additional calories.

When I needed something with a little more staying power—something I could send to school with Bea's lunch so she could dip berries into it—I graduated to Cool Whip Free, which didn't melt after being dispensed from its container. This preternatural tendency probably has something to do with the confection's synthetic composition. I confess I found its hardiness a little spooky. But it jazzed up Bea's lunch bag so much, enhancing the prospect of eating berries—*again*—while the kids sitting next to her scarfed down candy or snack bars. It wasn't a staple of her diet; she ate just a dollop of it every couple of days. And each tablespoon of this unmeltable substance had only 7.5 calories, so I welcomed it into my home. It served a purpose.

Cool Whip Free became part of a dessert I devised in which I plopped a spoonful of the stuff into a mini phyllo cup (17.5 calories each), with a juicy blackberry, pair of blueberries, or section of strawberry on top as a pretty and colorful garnish. I called these "mini fruit tarts," and they looked really cute and tasted pretty good. Sweets-averse David showed his typical lack of interest in them, but Jeff admitted they were decent. Most important, Bea liked them, and, perhaps absurdly, I was quite proud of them.

Late one afternoon, Bea and I decided to make a batch so that she could bring them in for a celebration they were having at school the next day. I knew there would be lots of tempting, fattening offerings available, and preferred Bea to have a lower-calorie option. We were out with Bea's friend and her mom, and we stopped in at the grocery store to get the necessary ingredients. Bea picked up the Cool Whip Free. I couldn't find the mini phyllo cups.

Time was ticking, and we still had to make these little tarts (admittedly quick, but time-consuming in volume enough for the class). With an inflexibility born of my intense focus on getting this task done, I couldn't imagine coming up with a similarly diet-friendly alternative at that point.

"Okay. We have to go to the other store," I decided. I was pretty sure they'd be in stock at the giant supermarket many blocks away.

I was trying to get Bea on board with the plan to leave her friend in order to pursue mini phyllo cups when the friend's mom intervened.

"What is it you guys are making?" she asked. She took the Cool Whip Free from Bea's hands and started selectively reading off the ingredients. "Water, corn syrup, hydrogenated vegetable oil, high-fructose corn syrup, artificial flavor, modified food starch, xanthan and guar gums, polysorbate 60, polysorbate 65, sorbitan monostearate, sodium hydroxide . . ."

"Okay, thanks," I said, allowing a hint of my annoyance to seep through my smile. I had an hour to concoct a low-calorie snack for Bea's entire class and didn't appreciate the health lecture.

"Bea, why would you want to eat all these chemicals?" she asked. She was being playful, but she was definitely trying to impart a nutrition lesson that I figured she felt I had failed to teach. Maybe she was even implying that she resented my foisting these unhealthful ingredients on her child, who was Bea's classmate and who would be present at the next day's event where my mini fruit tarts were to be served.

I said we had to check another store for the missing ingredient. I took Bea's hand and we left the supermarket for the judgment-free aisles of the other store, where we bought our mini phyllo cups, Cool Whip Free, and berries in peace.

I understood where my friend was coming from. And though I was irritated that she would try to make Bea (or me) feel bad about what we were eating while knowing full well that we were on this weight-loss program, I had to remember that just a few months before, I had not been that different from her. I had made food purchasing decisions based partially on the healthfulness of the product. If I could get something organic at roughly the same price as the non-organic, I chose the former. If there was a whole-grain version of something that looked about as tasty as the more processed variety, I went with the whole grains.

No doubt, processed foods are a worse choice nutritionally than whole foods. And I am not immune to concern about the possibility of long-term health risks associated with our population's consumption of preservatives and artificial sweeteners and coloring agents. I did not actively seek to add artificial ingredients and fat or sugar substitutes to my children's diets. But I also didn't shy away from them when they showed up in foods that made Bea's journey a bit easier and more kid friendly.

No normal child can entirely avoid being exposed to junk food. It would have been unrealistic to ask Bea to follow a diet devoid of carbs and processed foods. I mean, where would we have drawn the line on "processed" anyway? White rice? Grape jelly? Canned tuna? Hummus? It's hard to know, as an average consumer, when things really start to get ugly from an ingredients standpoint.

Based on our lifestyle, Jeff and I chose a weight-loss program that allowed Bea to eat everything in restrained amounts, because that was a way to teach her how to manage real-world eating for the long term. It would not have made sense to try to exclude the kinds of foods that a growing number of parents look down on as "bad" or "unhealthy."

Since beginning this diet, I had found my priorities shifting. Instead of looking for whole grains and organic ingredients, I now compared calorie content, fat grams, and portion sizes. I paid some attention to fiber, but only because I knew it would keep Bea fuller longer, and possibly aid in the process of getting the food out of her body once it was digested. The 80-calorie all-fruit frozen pops I had previously bought (and continued to buy for David) seemed hulking and ignorant compared with the slender 20-calorie sugar-free Popsicles I now purchased for Bea. I wasn't happy that the reduced calorie content also brought with it maltodextrin, aspartame, artificial flavors, red 40, yellow 6, and blue 1. But I accepted them because the snack better served the purposes of our larger goal.

In the stumbling-across-information-that-will-prove-your-own-hunch department, it was around this time that I found an article that had been published a few months earlier on CNN's website with the headline "Twinkie Diet Helps Nutrition Professor Lose 27 Pounds." It described the ten-week, 1,800-calorie-a-day junk food diet undertaken by Mark Haub, a professor of human nutrition at Kansas State University. He not only lost weight and body fat, his "bad" cholesterol went down, and his "good" cholesterol went up. He ate some healthful food and took vitamin supplements, but two-thirds of his calories came from snack cakes.

In the article, Haub was careful not to advocate this diet as any kind of model others should follow in the interest of health. It did, however, illustrate the importance of portion control and calorie reduction when seeking weight loss, and that fewer pounds on an overweight body will improve overall health. A spokeswoman for the American Dietetic Association was quoted in the article as saying, "When you lose weight . . . even if it's with packaged foods, generally you will see these markers [such as cholesterol and blood pressure] improve."

Haub also said that he didn't think dieters should seek a "total removal" of junk foods from their diets in favor of fruits and vegetables. "It may be healthy, but not realistic," he said. I loved this guy in that moment. I had lived by these tenets in my own life, and had, over the long haul, maintained a healthy weight. Bea had become obese on a healthful diet. Her father struggles with his weight, even though he almost never eats highly processed foods. This article confirmed my confidence in the proposition that it's better to lose weight by eating some junk food than to eat only healthy foods and be overweight.

Look, diet fads come and go, but there is no debate that someone who burns more calories than he takes in will lose weight. You can achieve that energy balance in any number of ways, through excluding certain food groups or increasing activity. But the bottom line is, if you want to lose weight, you're going to have to eat less. Calories matter.

But you shouldn't think I was completely cavalier regarding nutrients. My confidence in my choices was occasionally shaken. For example, one day I was looking up recipes I could make for Bea using my dependable Cool Whip Free, and I found a blog posting written by a seemingly un-crazy, un-sanctimonious person about how unhealthy this product was. She criticized its use of both corn syrup *and* high-fructose corn syrup as two of the top four ingredients, and then explained that what really made her throw out the tub forever was the presence of a small amount of partially hydrogenated vegetable oil, which contains trans fats.

She complained that Kraft indicates on the nutrition label via an asterisk that the amount is "negligible," and indeed, as the blogger explained via a link, if a product has less than 0.5 gram of trans fat, it can consider itself trans fat free even if it's technically not.

Now, I can't tell you what exactly trans fats are or what they do, but I know that everyone hates them, they're being banned by cities all over the place, and they have some negative impact on cholesterol. So, sure, I'm on board with avoiding them. They were, in fact, one of the few things our nutrition doctor told us we should never, ever eat. Whoa, okay then—out with the Cool Whip Free!

But wait . . . let's take another look at that food label. As it turns out, Cool Whip Free's fourth ingredient is "hydrogenated vegetable oil," not the partially hydrogenated kind the blogger cited. Awesome! Let's put that tub back into the freezer!

Not so fast. According to the Mayo Clinic, fully hydrogenated oil doesn't contain trans fat, but if a label says "hydrogenated vegetable oil," as my Cool Whip Free does, it "could mean" it contains trans fat. Um, so what exactly does that mean for my light frozen whipped topping?

I still don't know. My research did nothing but confuse me, and though I made no formal policy decision in response, I found that while I continued buying fat-free Reddi-wip whipped cream, my practice of buying Cool Whip Free ended, and with it, the era of the mini fruit tart and make-your-own fruit parfaits in Bea's lunch bag. The incident served to remind me of how utterly perplexing and misleading nutrition information can be for the average consumer trying to make informed and nutritious choices for her family.

Let me be clear: I am not going to stand up for processed foods and advocate that they must be a part of a well-balanced diet. However, there's no getting around the fact that they proved extremely useful in motivating Bea to stick with her program. Sugar substitutes help cut the calorie content of things my child likes to eat, so I sometimes bought foods that contained them. Bea's health issue is not one specifically proscribing the consumption of sodium or cholesterol or lactose. Her issue requires the avoidance of excess calories. So sometimes I chose a low-calorie Snackwells cookie, with all its additives and imitation sugars, over a more wholesome but higher-calorie oatmeal-raisin alternative because, ironically, it was a better health choice for Bea.

In case you weren't aware, that's a wildly controversial position. Having been on both sides of the opinion spectrum regarding healthful foods versus processed foods, I completely understand the repugnance some people feel about feeding junky food to kids. There's a reflexive judgment made about a parent with an overweight child when that child is seen eating junk food—even if that food, unbeknownst to the casual observer, has been carefully chosen for its lower calorie content and motivational properties.

On a playdate during one of those early weeks, I handed Bea her 100-calorie pack of yogurt-covered pretzels while her friend ate a Whole Foods apple cereal bar that, no question about it, was more nutritious than Bea's snack, but also was 40 percent more caloric.

"Does Bea want a cereal bar?" her friend's dad asked. "I have an extra one."

"No, thanks," I answered, in unison with Bea's resounding "Yes!"

"Bea, you have your snack," I reminded her.

A snapshot of the scene creates a discomfiting picture: the heavy kid eating the processed, packaged snack, and the thin kid eating the wholesome, Whole Foods–brand snack. The mother of the overweight kid stubbornly refuses the more healthful snack, insisting on the nutritionally inferior one. What does this portrait imply to the average person witnessing it? That each parent's chosen snack has contributed to his or her child's weight status. That if the fat kid's mom listened to the thin kid's dad, the fat kid might look more like the thin kid. But only a parent of a child who struggles with the scale knows how oversimplified that is.

This sort of moment occurs constantly for us. I can't defend nutritionally deficient low-calorie processed snacks against higher-calorie nutritious ones to anyone. I have a different gut reaction to seeing a parent give a child a packet of organic baked brown rice chips than I do to seeing one hand her kid a bag of Funyuns. I also have a different emotional response when I see an overweight kid eating a king-size Kit Kat, and when I see a thin kid eating a king-size Kit Kat. I just do. I knew there were societal judgments that went along with giving an overweight child processed snacks, because I was guilty of those judgments as well. But I had to ignore them.

Usually the parents who knew Bea and me well were the least judgmental. It was the moms I met at the playground or chatted with only occasionally at school who would pepper our discussions with sanctimony. If they overheard me refusing Bea a second serving of lunch, they'd mildly note that kids are still growing and suggest that I should let Bea eat if she was still hungry. They'd criticize the size or quality of Bea's snack, unaware that it was the result of a great deal of thought and planning.

"Do you know how bad that stuff is for her?" a fellow parent asked me upon seeing Bea bust open a package of miniature Oreo Cakesters I'd been delighted to come across in the supermarket. The comment was made in a friendly way, as though maybe I really didn't know and she could be helpful and clue me in.

"Well, it fits in her diet, and I want her to get to have some junk food like other kids," I answered.

"You should at least give her snacks that aren't processed," the woman suggested.

"Her health priority is eating less, not eating healthier," I said. And it sounded idiotic even to me.

I'm obviously no expert on natural eating, and I admit I don't know whether certain ingredients are to be sought out or avoided. (To wit: is soy lecithin a good thing or a bad thing? How about citric acid? I know omega-3 fatty acids are really healthy, but don't they *sound* like they wouldn't be?) However, it seemed impossible to me that all these organic foods peddled to kids (and their parents) were entirely free of anything bad.

It turns out that the USDA permits dozens of non-organic ingredients in processed products labeled "organic." Carrageenan—which has been linked to ulcers and gastrointestinal cancer—is in many popular brands of organic cottage cheese and soy milk. Brown rice syrup—which can contain high levels of arsenic—is used as a sweetener in some organic cereal bars.

I'm the last person to be holier-than-thou about food ingredients. I'm not deriding these chemicals or the products that contain them. I would happily eat an organic cereal bar (and now that I write about it, I sort of wish I were eating one right this minute), and I would feed one to my child. I'm just saying that making kids eat only organic food doesn't necessarily mean they're not also ingesting some questionable ingredients. And the messages we parents get about how to best nourish our kids are often perplexing and contradictory.

Ironically, I felt like a really good mom when I met Bea after school one day and gave her a 100-calorie three-pack of Hostess mini cream-filled cupcakes. As she ate them, another kid—one with no weight problem or dietary issues—saw her chomping on those little cupcakes and let out a jealous wail. A normal-weight kid who could eat whatever he wanted was jealous of Bea's snack! Yay, me!

What struck me as hypocritical was that even parents whose day-to-day food choices for their children are very healthful do generally relent sometimes, allowing indulgent birthday treats or occasional fast-food excesses. I don't know many parents who really refuse their children processed foods 100 percent of the time. So let us people with weight problems have our kicks where we can get them! Bea wanted so much to be "normal" that processed foods were a small price to pay to help her feel that way.

I'd get flak from the other side, too—parents who felt (as I do) that summer ice cream cones and cookie chasers to birthday party cake slices are an inalienable right of childhood, and that by putting any limitation on Bea's consumption of those items, I was being callous. No matter how much effort I expended tailoring Bea's weekly food plans to allow participation in classroom treats and social celebrations, there always seemed to be a parent who felt I was cutting Bea off one Twinkie short and, in doing so, curtailing her childhood joy.

There it is, plain and simple: I'm damned if I do, damned if I don't. Some might have looked down on me for "letting" Bea become overweight. But then they offered their scorn when I decided to do the only thing that science and medicine agree is the best treatment, the thing that will decisively reverse her problem: that is, put her on a diet. Of course, it's not just me and it's not always about food. A working mom is judged negatively for letting someone else raise her kids, but a stay-at-home mom is accused of sacrificing her self-worth and providing an outdated role model for her children. Let your kids watch TV or play video games, and you're rotting their brains. Refuse to let them do so, and you're an oversheltering tyrant. You can't win.

There are healthy children who eat junk food all day and are still healthy. There are also unhealthy children who eat only natural, organic fare and are, sad to say, still unhealthy. As I said earlier, some things are just genetic. Not everyone who gets lung cancer smokes, and not every smoker gets lung cancer. Since letting a child eat some processed food is not definitely going to doom him to ill health, I see no reason to systematically deprive my healthy kids of it.

But I wondered: Was defending my decisions about what she should eat worth suffering this social unease? Worth making friends feel uncomfortable? Worth making Bea the subject of a public debate? Should I have just kept my mouth shut and let Bea eat the socially appropriate food of the moment, be it the Niçoise salad, the M&Ms, the cookie, the ramen soup, the calorie-packed organic snack? If so, what effect would that have had on her willingness to accept the limits I set in the future? And what cumulative effect would those little allowances have had on her weight over time?

I wasn't going to allow us to find out.

CHAPTER 8

"I hate this doctor, and I want to punch her in the face," Bea declared.

We were sitting in the nutrition doctor's waiting room. We'd been on the program for a couple of months, and I felt things were generally going well. Bea and I had been sticking closely to the regimen and had both lost about five pounds. For me, that rate of loss was unprecedentedly slow, but for Bea, it seemed right and I was proud of her progress. And for a child with no concern for his weight, David had an impressive level of dedication to the program. He would often ask if something was "healthy" before he ate it, or ask me to guide him in a choice between two foods ("Which is more healthy, penne or spaghetti?"). He sometimes took the stairs to our fourth-floor apartment instead of the elevator, and once he even climbed a small ski slope in lieu of riding the "magic carpet" conveyor, for the express purpose of pleasing our nutrition doctor.

Yet they both passionately hated these appointments. I figured it was normal, and analogous to a patient/therapist relationship. The work is difficult, so sometimes it can be hard to like the person overseeing it. We take out our frustration with the process on the doctor.

"I like her," I replied.

"Well, I didn't hate her at first," Bea admitted. "But the appointments are starting to grow drearier and drearier and drearier."

She was putting it mildly, I think. Bea's and David's attitudes toward our weekly appointments had disintegrated from mild intolerance to downright contempt. If Bea didn't much like the doctor or the associate we'd met on our second visit, she—and I—were even less excited about the third member of the doctor's team, who met with us on occasional weeks. This third woman, while friendly and enthusiastic, made the appointments she led feel like a day at school with an inept substitute teacher. The nutrition lecture we were supposed to receive never came when she was in charge. She didn't provide concrete answers to the questions I asked about food choices or feeding strategies, instead tossing the query back into my court with a less-than-helpful, "Well, what do *you* think?"

When we met this third woman about a month into our visits, I could sense that Bea felt uneasy that yet another person was hearing our food-related problems, writing notes about the previous week's triumphs and stumbling blocks, discussing her weight, seeing what the scale said when she stepped on. It was weird to try to pick up the thread of our journey with three different people on alternating weeks. To not have one person who would follow our progress, know our history, and understand the family dynamic was decidedly awkward.

Check-ins with the nutrition doctor herself were always more productive. But even with her, there was an incident one afternoon that bothered me. On the way to the appointment—as always, at four o'clock on a Friday—the kids had eaten their snacks. David had a slice of pizza. Bea had a green-light-size bag of Cheetos and a banana. Afterward, she complained that she was starving.

I knew that the scale was waiting for her and that it would either reward or disappoint our efforts of the preceding week. Bea had, as ever, worked hard to stick to the program. There had been the daily arguments over desired snacks I refused to provide, portion sizes she deemed insufficient, or treats given out at school that she had neglected to mention in time for them to be deducted from her after-school snack. But she had been a trouper, and I knew her willingness to adhere to the program wouldn't continue for long without the satisfaction of seeing a decrease in her weight. If she had another snack—even a piece of fruit—we were adding water weight that was going to cloud the results.

"Please, Mommy, I'm starving!" she pleaded.

We had arrived at the nutrition doctor's office building early. I couldn't deflect the request with the "we're running late" argument. We had plenty of time to spare to get something to eat.

"Can't you just wait until after the appointment?" I asked Bea. "Twenty minutes? Then I'll get you something?"

"No. I'm *starving*!" she implored me.

I felt deeply torn. My child was in distress, and it was within my power to help her, but I was withholding relief because I wanted her to have a gratifying weigh-in a few minutes later. It felt heartless, but was it so ridiculous to want to get an accurate and encouraging read on her weight? There was one occasion a week on which we could gauge how we were doing and be reminded that all our hard work was leading us steadily to lower weight and better health. Giving in on a snack now meant jeopardizing our weekly affirmation that we were making progress. I saw Bea's face as she stepped on the scale every week. I knew that what it said mattered to her. Was its readout this week important enough to ask her to hold out another half hour? To me, absolutely. To her? Obviously not.

I gave in. We popped into a deli across the street from the office. I was happy to see they had a large array of cut-up fresh fruit. David selected a container of mango. Bea opted for a large container of watermelon.

It was probably about two or three cups of watermelon—maybe twelve ounces. Which is three-quarters of a pound on the scale. It's not fat weight, it's water weight. But if you step onto a scale holding a box of watermelon, you're going to weigh more than if you aren't holding the watermelon. Putting the fruit in your stomach is just another way of carrying that weight. That's just physics.

After Bea polished off the watermelon, the nutrition doctor came out to greet us. She first measured both kids to see if they had grown—their height was unchanged—and then put Bea on the scale.

"She just had some watermelon," I blurted out as the numbers settled on the scale. Bea's weight had gone up about half a pound.

"We're going in the wrong direction," the nutrition doctor said, not unkindly.

"I think it was the watermelon," I noted.

We took our seats.

"So what happened this week?" the doctor asked.

Now, it's very possible that those were the words she used to start every appointment. But this week I took it as an accusation.

"Nothing happened this week," I snapped. "Bea's been great.

She was just really, really hungry, so she just had a giant thing of watermelon. That's why it looks like she gained weight."

Bea was sitting quietly in her seat, looking downcast. I couldn't bear for her to think her efforts weren't being acknowledged, that her dedication was being questioned.

"You know, Bea and I have been talking about how the scale isn't always going to go down every week," I continued. "That sometimes it will go up because of how she eats, or sometimes it will just go up for no reason, and that that's part of the process, and she shouldn't feel bad about it. Can you maybe talk a little bit about that?"

As the nutrition doctor explained the vagaries of body weight, I continued to interpret her every word as a response to some sort of presumed weight gain. Maybe I'm projecting here, but I felt like she was telling Bea not to worry about the fact that she had overeaten this week and gained weight. It was bound to happen. It was part of the process. From Bea's expression, she seemed not quite chastened but definitely disappointed.

I, however, was sure she hadn't actually gained weight.

As the appointment wound down, I asked the doctor point-blank how much weight Bea had to lose before she reached a healthy weight. I had been eager to know, of course, but had resisted asking because I knew it wasn't a politically correct question. I'm not supposed to be focused on pounds, first of all, but rather the more obscure metric of BMI. And I felt like I was supposed to perpetuate some kind of modern charade that even though they weighed her every Friday, the scale didn't matter—that how we felt, how our clothes fit, and how many miles we could run were the true barometers of physical health.

But I'm extremely number-focused. To me, weight *was* numbers: what the scale said, how many pounds I wanted to lose, how many calories I could eat. I know I'm never going to look like a supermodel. So I have to take the subjectivity out of it, just pick a number that I think is attainable and maintainable, and go for that.

As for Bea, I wasn't trying to make her slender. That wasn't my job. I just needed her to be healthy. So I wanted to know where that category began for her. I was concerned that, without a number as my finish line, I wouldn't know when to stop, and I'd end up trying to make her thin instead of just not overweight. Or that I'd get tired of the process, and give up before we'd gotten to a truly healthy weight. I was fine with replacing calories with "green lights," but the lack of a concrete, numeric goal for Bea's weight made it difficult for me to grasp what we were in for. I wanted some kind of understanding of where we needed to end up.

The nutrition doctor explained that she doesn't like to talk about numbers. People become too fixated on them, she said. And anyway, with kids, they're always growing and so the goal is constantly moving. She told me that it was better to concentrate on making positive changes and not think so much about the numbers. She was absolutely right. I totally got it. I still couldn't stand it.

"Makes sense," I said. "I guess I just wanted a sense of how long a road we should expect this to be."

She looked down at her chart and waited until Bea was looking away before catching my eye conspiratorially. She mouthed one word to me: "Long."

It was a lighthearted way of communicating a difficult piece of news, and I wished at that moment that my husband were there to help provide some support and levity. When Jeff used to come to these visits with us, we'd sit in the waiting room with me grumpily deflecting the kids' demands that we go home and never come back, and he was able to lighten the mood by cracking just the right joke. He was able to add just enough silliness to get us through with a smile. Just by his being there, the appointments felt a little bit like special occasions.

But we'd excused Jeff from these appointments after the first few weeks. I felt it was ridiculous for him to leave work early every single Friday so he could sit with us for twenty minutes in the nutrition doctor's office. It was causing too much upheaval to his schedule, and other than comic relief, he wasn't really contributing all that much to our time there. We'd agreed I'd take the kids on my own.

Jeff remained engaged in Bea's progress and supportive of the plan we'd adopted, but around the same time he stopped coming to the appointments, he also stopped following the diet himself.

After we'd been on the program for a week, he had stepped on the scale at home and he was heavier than he'd been at our initial weigh-in at the nutrition doctor's office. He was not pleased.

"It's the fruit," he said, blaming the program's permitted late-night binges on grapes and oranges for the apparent weight gain.

At that time, Bea had taken off almost a pound. I didn't want Jeff's disappointment to throw us off course. "Give it a little more time," I said.

"It's the fruit," he said definitively.

He wasn't explicitly giving up, but he did not follow up that reproach with a plan. I felt pressure to keep him on board, but I had nothing constructive to suggest. I just hoped he'd hang in there and that results would be forthcoming. But after another week or so, even though the scale did indeed start heading downward, he gave up counting his traffic lights.

Jeff and I often approach parenting as a divide-and-conquer proposition. For example, I have never once cut my children's nails. It's just something that he does, so I don't even think about it. Now, surely Bea's health and diet are more important and complicated than her nails. So it made sense that Jeff had been an integral part of acknowledging her issue and setting the family off on a path to address it. But in terms of the day-to-day management, he felt confident that if I had things under control, he didn't need to be very involved.

I didn't expect otherwise. But it did sometimes get problematic.

For example, Jeff had no idea how many green lights Bea was allocated at any given meal. And if he was, say, making her a pork chop, I'd have to remind him to weigh it, look up the calories in an ounce of pork, and do the math. Only then would he realize that he needed to cut the chop in half for it to be the right size for Bea.

"I don't translate food into calories, and certainly not into 'green lights,'" he explained. "It's a pork chop. It's protein, it's good, it's 'the other white meat.' That can't be bad."

But too much of a good thing could be bad. He himself had greeted our doctor's permissiveness of fruit with much suspicion. And I couldn't disagree with him. I still very strongly suspected that the amount one ate, more so than what one ate, was of paramount importance to weight. While the Atkins revolution had taken an impressively persuasive stab at my long-held axiom—claiming as it did that you could basically eat any caloric amount of proteins and fats as long as you eliminated carbohydrates—I was still fearful of any program that allowed unlimited consumption of anything, even fruit.

The ability to offer Bea fruits or vegetables to eat at any time was useful, however. I appreciated having an option to provide when Bea complained of being hungry right after finishing lunch, or having something with which to answer David's demand for a snack right before bed. But Bea's appetite for fruits and vegetables—mostly fruits—was seemingly endless. She could put away several bananas in one sitting. At around 100 calories each, that's not nothing. And they weren't exactly carb-free. Although I understood we were supposed to care less about the carbohydrates in fresh fruit than about the ones in chocolate cake, hadn't Dr. Atkins revealed to us how sinister most fruits could be? That even though they have vitamins and fiber, they're otherwise basically just sugar delivery mechanisms? So were fruits good or bad? It was hard to sort out the conflicting wisdom about these kinds of things.

Even oranges and apples had seventy to eighty calories each. And on more than one occasion I realized that Bea had eaten five servings of fruit between dinner and bedtime. I permitted it, because the nutrition doctor said it was okay, and because Bea was being so amazingly compliant about the reduction in food in other areas. But it was worthy of notice. Shouldn't I be teaching her moderation, even where healthful foods were involved? And she wasn't the only one liberated by the all-you-can-eat fruit rule: One weekend morning at a friend's house, Bea, David, and I collectively managed to put away two pounds of strawberries over the course of a leisurely brunch. We could really pack it in.

One night, Bea herself acknowledged that she had taken too much advantage of the all-fruit-you-can eat policy.

"I think I just ate too many apples," she admitted. "And it makes me feel stuffed. And it makes me feel like I overate, even though I didn't."

I asked her what that feeling was like emotionally for her.

"I feel unhealthy," she said. "Because I feel like when you stuff yourself, it's not good for you. Even when the food is good for you, it's not good to stuff yourself every night because you don't feel well in the morning and you don't want to go places and do anything. It's better to be nice, healthy, quick—like quick to do things, ready to do things."

I was pleased by Bea's take. She wasn't accusing herself of having eaten something "bad," and her regret was not "Now I feel fat" but "Now I don't feel so well, and I'm not in the mood to do other things that are part of life." The lesson was certainly superior to how I'd learned restraint. It was better to feel a little stuffed from apples than to suffer crushing guilt after a bonanza donut binge.

CHAPTER 9

My friend does a funny riff on how women in her social circle act around the cake at a party. She describes how they stalk around it for a while, checking it out, seeing who else is eating it. They visit it a couple of times, often striking up a conversation with another woman about how good it looks, and whether they should try it. Those who do dig in often do so from a position of apology or explanation: how they're going to pay for it later by going to the gym or skipping dessert for the next few days, but it's worth it. And every bite they take seems to tell a self-conscious story of longing, gratification, and guilt. Then of course, there's the hostess's panic when the party winds down and she confronts the thought of being alone in the house with the leftovers. She entreats her guests to have another slice, to take some home—anything to avoid being left alone with it, like the cake is an axe murderer or something.

Splurging on fattening food is an emotionally mixed proposition for most women. Now that cake was no longer the staple food it had been in my younger years, when I had happily sacrificed healthful fare to allow for it, I shared the popular feelings of anxiety around such excess. But I wanted Bea to understand that it's not realistic or even ideal to turn down a slice of her aunt's wedding cake even though we had already eaten the big steak and cheesy potatoes we'd been served for dinner. Sometimes—and only on rare and truly special occasions (a wedding being both)—I let us both go for it. And I would always take a moment to make sure Bea was mindful that it was okay to do so once in a while.

But I was uneasy with the program's permissiveness of certain foods in unlimited amounts—fat-free cheese, tomato juice, edamame, sugar-free Jell-O. As with the fruit, I felt that not curtailing the consumption of these foods was teaching a confusing lesson about the need for moderation. I couldn't decide whether the benefit of letting Bea have unfettered access to these things justified the abandon with which she sometimes approached them.

On one of the weeks when the nutrition doctor herself met with us, she led a discussion about being aware of how much we're eating, even if it's healthful food. She told of a patient who ate low-fat cheese on reduced-calorie bread, but too many slices of each. This patient had skim milk and healthful cereal for breakfast, but too many cups. You get the picture. The point was, just because something is low-fat, low-calorie, or "healthful" does not mean it can't make you gain weight.

This, in a nutshell, was Jeff's problem. While my weight gains always had obvious sources in sugar, fat, and carbs, he actually loved and preferred healthful food. But volume was his main issue: tomatoes and cucumbers drizzled in tablespoons of olive oil, or wheat crisps slathered with feta cheese, or something involving a lot of chickpeas or nuts. There was no obviously villainous food going into his body, but there was a lot of it, and many of his very nutritious choices were absolutely packed with calories.

I am aware of the irony that things such as hummus and olives made me nervous while I felt perfectly comfortable with sugar-free Jell-O. However, I reserved the right to call the shots and didn't initially extend this generosity of spirit to soda.

I don't like soda. Never did. As a kid, I found the carbonation unpleasant and the taste too syrupy. Regardless, I often drank diet soda, because it has no calories, occasionally water gets boring, and my preferred black iced tea is not always available. But I had never let my kids have soda. It seemed the pinnacle of completely unnatural, nutritionless, chemically engineered garbage. When other parents served their kids Coke, I was super judgmental. Caffeine, sugar, carbonation—why not just give them Red Bulls? Jeff and I let Bea have club soda, and that was it.

But one night we were out to dinner with Bea and David's cousins, and they ordered Shirley Temples. Turning to Bea and David, the waiter said innocently, "Same for you?" I panicked. Not merely a glass of soda, but an additional shot of sugary grenadine and a maraschino cherry, just to rub it in?

David declined, requesting an orange juice instead. Soda is one of the many sweets he doesn't care for. But before Bea could answer the waiter, I jumped in and tried to steer things to a "better" place:

"Would you like a Diet Coke?" I asked. The words felt strange in my mouth. Offering soda was weird enough; offering diet soda to a child seemed downright perverse.

"I want a Shirley Temple," Bea said.

"You can't have a Shirley Temple," I said gently. "How about a club soda with a little splash of cranberry juice?" To tell you the truth, even offering the splash of cranberry juice felt like a concession, but we were under pressure. The waiter stood by expectantly.

"No. A Shirley Temple," Bea insisted.

"Bea, you can't," I replied. I laid out her options: "Diet Coke or club soda with cranberry juice?"

"Diet Coke," she grumbled.

And from then on I let her order a diet soda any time we went out to dinner. I almost forgot how grotesque I had found the practice when other parents had done it before Bea started this diet. It wasn't just that I wanted Bea to have a little calorie-free indulgence when we went out. A diet soda came to seem like a legitimately superior choice when compared with the sugary Shirley Temples and apple juices readily offered to kids in restaurants. I know how obscene it seems to health-conscious moms, but to cover up the lack of orange juice, milk, and smoothies in Bea's life, I started adding six-packs of diet soda to my grocery lists.

And so we trudged along, my days mired in the monotony of maintaining a steady nutritional rhythm for each member of the family. Every morning Bea and I ate every crumb of our tiny breakfasts, while David got a larger portion but didn't finish it. Each child headed off to school with a packed lunch containing about 100–150 calories of protein, 50–100 calories of carbohydrate, about fifty calories of dairy, and lots of fresh fruits and vegetables, with an added Rice Krispies Treat tucked into David's lunch box.

Every night I continued to make two dinners: a bland protein with large side dishes of pasta and vegetables for David, and a carefully curated, prepared, and portion-controlled dish for me and Bea, with my husband eating the same thing in double the amount.

Every week we examined our schedule and strategized about how to avoid any potential stumbling blocks. Over and over again.

If it sounds like I did little else but plan and execute my family's meals during this year, that's sort of true. Yes, I worked and socialized and ran my household and had fun with my husband and kids. But my priority was Bea's diet, and in the back of my mind, her needs influenced every decision. Kids need to be fed five or six times a day. It's a rare plan that can be made for an activity, a vacation, a social visit, or even a simple day at home that doesn't at some point involve food. Bea's diet needed to be a constant consideration.

I tried to do most of this sort of planning behind the scenes, but I also brought Bea into the process so that she'd learn how to deal with food on her own. I tried to ensure that the decision making would be fun for her; we both did quite like talking about food. But I couldn't imagine many other seven-year-olds were looking at restaurant menus online before going out to dinner, or brainstorming ideas for what they could bring to a class potluck that wouldn't put too big a dent in their day's allotment of calories. I wished Bea didn't have the burden of always having to think about making "smart" or "good" choices, or sacrificing one desired food in order to enjoy another.

"I know doing this is annoying," I told her one afternoon as we argued over what she'd choose to eat that night at a restaurant whose menu we were perusing.

"That's my life. It's always going to be my life, and I can't change it," she sighed. "It's something I have to deal with."

Oh, my. "Does it make you sad?" I asked. I worried all the time that the requirements of this endeavor would damage my relationship with Bea. With food so prevalent in our lives, I felt like I was forever raising an eyebrow, questioning a choice, avoiding a tricky eating environment. Bea, in addition to being a great kid, is also just a fun person to hang out with. Food had so often been part of the enjoyment of our special time together. What was going to happen now that our periodic giddy trips to the bakery for a cupcake had to become carefully orchestrated occurrences? When seeing a movie together no longer involved sharing a big bag of buttery popcorn? When we couldn't spontaneously decide on a lazy Sunday afternoon to catch up with each other while baking chocolate chip cookies?

Was every restaurant dinner going to be blemished by an argument over the bread basket? Would every birthday party be made tense by a negotiation at the dessert table? Would every description of a school event she participated in devolve into an interrogation about what she ate?

Considering that litany also made me question our very lifestyle. Why is food involved in so many of our social events and recreational outings? Maybe the problem wasn't just how we approached food in these situations but also that food was a part of them in the first place. I wondered if we were going to have to start looking at every event anew, figuring out ways to exclude food from it when eating had been an anticipated and enjoyed part of it previously. Maybe, instead of bringing lower-calorie food to a picnic in the park, we should just go to the park to play and *not have the picnic at all.* It was a whole new way of thinking, and it seemed a big shift to make.

I was proud of the relationship I'd built with Bea. I felt I had found a good balance of mothering and friendship, of leadership and silliness. I treasured our time together. I was scared that the role I'd now taken on had shifted the dynamic. Planning was replacing spontaneity. Fun was sometimes pushed out in favor of enforcement.

I was troubled by that change. I dearly hoped that what I believed in my heart—that the sacrifices we were making now would be far outweighed by the long-term benefits to Bea's health and happiness—was true. Even if this process couldn't ensure that Bea would enjoy a healthy relationship to food in the future, at least we were talking about it in a frank and consistent way. While Bea certainly found my impositions annoying, I did not feel she loved me less for it. We still found ways to laugh and be close and spend special time together. There were just a lot fewer calories involved.

"It may actually sound sad, but it's my life, you know?" Bea said. "Once you start going on a diet, it makes you feel great, but inside you know that you're different from other people. And you'll never be able to change that."

Being like everyone else was important to Bea, as it is to most kids. And the hardest part of the diet for her was that it made her feel different. But she also knew that being heavy made her feel different, too. So while these discussions seemed to steal some of her innocence, making her think and act like an adult with a weight problem, we both hoped that doing so would save her from actually becoming that person.

For both Bea and me, the first thing that came to mind when we thought of a birthday party was cake. When we contemplated a visit to a new city, what we looked forward to was not the sights, not the shopping, not the hotel or the people, but the food. A visit to our friends' house in the country? They always have that awesome natural peanut butter. That was our essential nature, and wasn't going to change easily, if ever. It was important to plan our activities in such a way that we could accommodate some of the delicacies that were always on our minds, yet not allow them to be the central focus.

With that in mind, I prepared for our first big family vacation since we'd started the diet. And though to our family a "big" vacation is all of four days, we were going to a resort in Mexico where we'd be eating all of our meals out. I was nervous. I had the hotel send me their restaurant menus in advance, and mentally planned out our meals.

As is my habit, I was trying, and failing, to pre-lose some weight before the trip. The idea, always, was that I'd drop a few pounds so I could enjoy the food at my destination and come back at a normal-ish weight. I don't think I've ever really succeeded in achieving this goal, but I always try. Bea's weight hadn't gone down much the week before we left, either. I would have to be vigilant on our vacation.

We'd been to this resort before, and I knew what was likely to happen. We would have a big breakfast at the hotel buffet, then we'd get hungry around the pool midmorning and order a snack. Then we wouldn't be hungry for lunch until about 2:00 p.m. But we'd need another small snack at around five, and then have dinner at seven-thirty or so. Not only were these quick little poolside or beach snacks neither quick nor small (we'd end up sharing a big cheesy quesadilla and chicken fingers, or getting a sandwich that came with lots of fries), they were also quite expensive. So my hope was that this time I could figure out a way to cut costs *and* calories.

The breakfast buffet was included with our room rate, so we went there every morning. Bea and I chose our breakfast very carefully—it was hard with all those amazing choices, including Mexican dishes and a table full of sweet baked goods, along with the usual bagels, cereals, eggs, and sausage. Bea usually chose a small bagel with peanut butter, and I had a couple of poached eggs and tomatoes. I asked for some to-go containers, which I loaded up with fruit (for Bea) and pigs in blankets (for David). That was our midmorning snack. We then had a proper but light lunch, and in the afternoon we'd have a snack from a stash of granola bars and snack packs I'd brought in my suitcase from New York, plus a plum or apple from the in-room fruit bowl they refilled every day. Then we'd try to have a reasonable dinner, even though that was complicated by the fact that Bea discovered the existence of these little fried tortilla sandwiches called pork panuchas and wanted to order them every day (fortunately, they came in a reasonable appetizer size).

In this way, we were able to keep pretty much on track. Of course, there were obstacles. Homemade mango pops, pineapple smoothies, and other fruity frozen treats were handed out periodically at the pool. And one night was my birthday, so my husband arranged for dinner on the beach with bonfire s'mores and a smiley-face cake delivered to our room afterward (we each had a tiny slice, and then we sent the cake away with the housekeeping staff). I let Bea have all of it without so much as a significant glance.

My inflexibility at breakfast and strategizing around snacks made it possible for us to enjoy these excesses. And that was kind of the point: because I was willing to be the unyielding enforcer every meal of every day, we could sip a smoothie at the pool or have unforeseen s'mores on the beach. Whenever I questioned my own insistence on counting every calorie, tracking every bite, this reality would soon rear its head. Hardly a day in life goes by without some unexpected food being proffered. It was important that I maintain a Draconian level of rigidity so that we could sometimes say yes to these little surprises.

For people like me, Jeff, and Bea, the enjoyment of food is a big part of what vacation—and life—is all about.

CHAPTER 10

I had found that while Jeff supported the general initiative of helping Bea get healthy, he was considerably less rigorous than I was with the execution. If it seemed fun to nibble on a few french fries at lunch with Bea, or take her for frozen yogurt on a Saturday afternoon, he did it.

I appreciated that he got her yogurt instead of ice cream, but not when she'd already had her afternoon snack. And it's good that they only ate a few fries (if their unwavering account is to be trusted), but they really should have had zero.

Our opposing roles in this effort—Mom as the heavy, Dad as the fun guy—were characteristic of our general parenting personas. We were usually on the same page overall, but we went about getting there very differently. As two stubbornly opinionated people, we had arguments that were always, as my husband put it, "only about things that were never going to change." I wasn't about to loosen up. He wasn't going to stress himself out. I thought an extra frozen yogurt was a big setback. He thought it was a useful break from the stringency of Bea's diet.

It was easy for me to get annoyed with what I often saw as his hindrance of our progress. But if I think about it in a calm moment, I suppose that sort of balance is helpful for our kids, and even for the dieting process. In the same way that I see value in letting Bea have some nutritionally deficient but fun treat every day to stay motivated, Jeff's more permissive approach to eating, as long as it wasn't frequent or excessive, was probably a good thing for her, too. He let me oversee the kids' eating my way when they were on my watch, even when he felt I was sometimes too strict. So I returned the favor when it was his turn to feed them. It wasn't that often, in any case.

But one area in which my husband and I do not at all see eye to eye is with regard to the utility of exercise. He wakes up an hour early four times a week and works out at the gym, while I sleep. He has exercise clothes and gadgets, whereas I honestly don't even own a pair of sneakers. The fact that it has taken me this long to talk at any length about exercise is reflective of my general attitude toward it—which is that it is hugely overrated as a tool in weight loss.

I know that this attitude often makes jaws drop in shock at my ignorance, but hear me out. There are three reasons I can think of why people work out: for their health (improving their cardiovascular functioning, reducing risk of heart disease, prolonging life span), for fitness (being able to lift a suitcase into a car trunk, carry around a small child, take the stairs, run to catch a bus, ride a bike for fun), and for weight loss (burning calories and fat in the expectation that it will lower one's body mass).

Let's start with the first one. I'm in favor of exercising for health. If someone has health problems such as heart disease, I can see that exercise would be a good thing. I do think it is possible to be healthy without exercise if you're genetically lucky. My grandmother Beatrice lived until she was 106, and you know she wasn't jogging or playing soccer during the entirety of the 1900s and early 2000s.

I am not a great role model in that department. I have a sedentary career, am terrible at sports, and find gyms deathly boring. Other than brisk daily walking—to the extent that it is convenient as I go about the execution of my errands and parental obligations—I do no formal exercise. Perhaps wrongly, I believe that my fortunate genetics and clean bill of health exempt me from the requirement of exercising for the sake of overall wellness or optimizing my life span.

Then there's physical fitness. In that department, too, I believe genetics has a hand. I believe that, with an inordinate amount of effort and time, I could train to, say, run several miles—slowly. Or do many repetitions of sit-ups. But that it would be more difficult for me than for someone more naturally inclined toward that kind of activity.

I do wish I were more physically fit—able to, say run the three blocks to meet Bea's school bus without stopping or more easily take the stairs in the event of an electrical outage. But the effort-benefit ratio does not make for a compelling argument to exercise for this purpose, given how much I hate it. So I don't. I'm strong enough to climb up the subway steps, to haul a suitcase, and to carry my children to bed when they fall asleep on the couch. Other than that, I make sure I'm on time for Bea's bus, and I hope for the best for the power grid.

I truly believe it is important for my children to exercise for their overall health and to do so in order to be physically fit—to be able to lift things, and run, and climb. So in my most do-as-I-say-not-as-I-do bit of parenting hypocrisy, I seek out physical activity for them, in order to instill the habit and give them the advantages that exercise can bring.

But as for exercise as an important tool in weight loss—I just cannot get on board.

Lack of exercise is one of the lifestyle deficiencies experts invoke to explain why we are getting fatter. Our bodies, the argument goes, evolved with the expectation that our survival would depend on a much higher level of activity in our daily lives than our current existence affords. But that explanation may be a red herring. In 2012, Herman Pontzer, an assistant professor of anthropology at Hunter College, reported some findings in *The New York Times* about the extent to which our sedentary lifestyles are to blame for the obesity epidemic. He studied the modern-day Hadza people of Tanzania, who still maintain a hunter-gatherer lifestyle. He found they burn the same number of calories per day as modern Americans do.

How can that be? Pontzer posits that our bodies adapt to account for our energy demands. "If we push our bodies hard enough, we can increase our energy expenditure, at least in the short term," Pontzer wrote. "But . . . our bodies adapt to our daily routines and find ways to keep overall energy expenditure in check." Our bodies evolved to compensate for increased levels of exertion.

The upshot: "We're getting fat because we eat too much, not because we're sedentary," Pontzer believes. And he agrees with me that while "physical activity is very important for maintaining physical and mental health . . . we aren't going to Jazzercise our way out of the obesity epidemic."

Let me acknowledge that I know there are people with more active lifestyles than mine, who burn more calories every day than I do, and who therefore can eat more. A waitress, a nurse, a kids' gymnastics coach—sure. There are also people who are super active in their leisure time, and they're in that same category. I have a friend who lives in the country, and when we go visit her for a weekend, I see that she is moving all day: tennis in the morning, a bike ride into town before lunch, a hike with her kids in the afternoon, et cetera. In the short term, that is going to affect what she can eat. These are people whose normal lives are different from mine because they engage in sustained activity for many hours per day. I'm never going to be like them, professionally or personally.

But let's talk about working out—the kind of forced, regular, discrete periods of exercise that people do in order to burn more calories, like jogging, riding a stationary bike, or going to a gym. I have periodically tried to integrate exercise into my weight-loss efforts. In high school when I joined Jack LaLanne, and fifteen years later at the New York City gym I tried out with my husband, I truly committed to going. I showed up several times a week to do circuit training, take aerobics or yoga classes, and hit the treadmill or rowing machine. Each time I gave it a real commitment for a full year.

My time at the gym may have made a difference—maybe I was slightly less out of breath upon rushing to the subway for work, or I could carry my handbag around with marginally less arm fatigue—but if so, the benefit was minuscule. And with all the effort I was expending, I was maybe burning 300 or 400 calories at each visit. Do you realize how quickly I can eat 400 calories? Exactly the number of seconds it takes to dip a soupspoon into a jar of peanut butter a few times. Do you know how willing I am to keep the lid on the peanut butter jar if it means saving the cost and effort of going to the gym, not to mention avoiding my deep dislike of every minute I spend there?

Then there's the fact that with increased exertion comes the need for increased caloric intake. So you're basically forced to compensate for your burned calories by eating more food than you otherwise would. I tried to challenge this theory by combining calorie cutting with increased exercise—the activities would seem to go hand in hand for a dieter—and the results were not good. It turns out that it's not ideal to go to the gym and hit the treadmill strenuously after work if you ate only a salad for lunch. I found that out the hard way, when I needed to be assisted out of my gym by a staff member after getting dizzy on the treadmill. But if you're going to have to bulk up on calories in order to have the energy to work out, what's the point, from a weight loss perspective?

I did not renew those gym memberships once they expired. And I stand by my belief that while I'd be in better shape in terms of muscle tone and cardiovascular fitness were I engaged in regular physical exercise, I wouldn't be substantially thinner.

Now, certainly, I have become skilled at finding evidence—anecdotal and otherwise—to support whatever theories about diet and exercise promote my personal worldview. But I've also tested these theories for decades, and I stick to what works. If exercise reliably made me drop weight, I'd make myself do it even though I hate it. If junk food in small quantities made me fatter, I'd avoid it. I am practical. I will do something faithfully, even if it makes me deeply unpopular with my own family, if it produces results. I focus my willpower where it will make a difference.

As it happens, my crackpot theories sometimes end up being affirmed by the scientific community. My anecdotal evidence about the pointlessness of working out for the purpose of weight reduction was bolstered in 2009 by a *Time* magazine article that confirmed that while exercise is useful in maintaining weight loss, it does not help people lose weight. It quoted Eric Ravussin, chair in diabetes and metabolism at Louisiana State University and, according to the article, a prominent exercise researcher. He said, "In general, for weight loss, exercise is pretty useless." It noted that exercise stimulates hunger, causes us to eat more, and "may even be making it harder" to lose weight. See?

Okay, so maybe the Internet makes it easy for anyone to buttress even the most obscure arguments with "scientific" support. There are certainly studies and articles I could cite whose findings are contrary to these. Maybe I'm only seeing what I'm looking for. But before you discard my theories, take a minute to consider them. Our cultural pattern is that we are all lemmings when it comes to the latest diet dogma, and then five years later that advice gets debunked and there's a new gospel. So I think it's fair to develop our own principles based on our personal anecdotal experience and gut feelings.

And while exercise has this squeaky-clean image, it can be a sensitive area for overweight kids. The fat kid being chosen last for team sports is a depressing cultural trope for a reason. Physical activity can be downright embarrassing for those not skilled at it. I recall watching TV with Bea one night when we flipped past an episode of *The Biggest Loser,* a show in which obese people compete to lose weight. As we watched the military-style exertion, humiliation, and deprivation to which the contestants are subjected, we happened upon a scene that I expect occurs in some incarnation each season. In it, an extremely overweight woman was being berated by a trainer at a gym, forced to do push-ups until she literally collapsed into tears.

I have to assume this poor woman on TV knew what she was in for when she signed on to a reality fitness show, but if that were me, I would feel utterly demoralized, as if I were a gross, out-of-shape pig who can't even do four push-ups without failing. Did the few minutes the trainer spent torturing her into a physical and mental breakdown really burn a lot of calories or give her a good idea of how to become more active?

Granted, this is not a normal, everyday exercise session. Most real-world workouts are more gentle, and I would hope most physical trainers are more emotionally supportive. But the popularity of drill-sergeant workout DVDs and the bumper crop of training gyms with "boot camp" in their names illustrate that many people think tougher is better when it comes to working out, and that the fatter and weaker you are, the more you would benefit from having someone kick your butt into better shape.

But to my mind, it would have made more sense for the TV trainer to take the woman on a slow stroll around the neighborhood, or maybe window shopping. She would have burned a lot more calories, seen how exercise could be not unpleasantly integrated into her daily routine, and not felt like a disgusting failure. But I realize that doesn't make good television.

I am pretty permissive when it comes to what appears on the television in my home. Since the age of two, my kids have watched *SpongeBob SquarePants,* which I acknowledge has taught them more synonyms for *idiot* than any other source. And if they crawl into my bed late at night, they're often treated to an episode of *The Daily Show,* even though I know Bea and David no longer accept my explanation that the bleeping noise covers up Jon Stewart's fondness for saying the word *stupid* a lot. But that night I disgustedly changed the channel away from *The Biggest Loser,* unable to watch—or to let Bea watch—that overweight woman's indignity and risk having Bea think that that sort of self-mortification was what fat people have to go through in order to become healthy.

While David was prone to run and jump around a lot, that just wasn't in Bea's nature. But we live in New York City. We walk a lot. Bea's young childhood had been filled with creative movement classes, multi-sports classes, swimming lessons, and dance. But we aren't exactly a sporty family, and my husband was the only one who engaged in exercise for exercise's sake. I wasn't about to force Bea to go jogging around our building or do jumping jacks in our apartment.

Bea was taking a gymnastics class once a week, and attending physical education classes at school and playing outside during recess. The nutrition doctor explained that wasn't enough. The Centers for Disease Control and Prevention recommend kids get sixty minutes of physical activity every day. According to a study of third graders conducted by The National Institute of Child Health and Human Development, in-school PE classes provide an average of only twenty-five minutes of activity per *week* to each child. We'd have to find a fun physical activity that Bea could do regularly, and enjoy.

I knew it was important for me to set aside my strongly held belief about the futility of exercise for weight loss and see to it that Bea had more activity in her schedule. One day Bea suggested she might be interested in taking karate. I went on the Internet and lucked into finding a traditional Japanese karate dojo right around the corner from our apartment.

We went one Saturday morning, and it was perfect. The place was a bright, minimalist studio, and the sensei who ran it was like a Hollywood version of the ideal karate instructor: firm but kind, disciplined and encouraging, serious but with a subtle sense of humor.

And Bea loved it instantly. Maybe it was the fact that it didn't require more aerobic capacity or coordination than she has, so she didn't feel like a moron doing it, as I so often did when I'd drop in on some random spin class with a friend. There was also an academic component to it, perfecting the movements in each kata and memorizing the Japanese and English names of each stance, block, strike, punch, and kick. The clear benchmarks for progress and graduation to a new belt level—with the stripe of colored tape applied to the old belt when promotion was imminent, and a formal and very real test to pass before getting that new belt—also appealed to her.

Here, at last, was perhaps a sport—an exercise, some movement—that she would embrace and that I could stand. She agreed to go at least twice a week. We joined the dojo. I finally felt good that, between gymnastics and karate, Bea was getting formal regular exercise a few times a week.

I definitely considered that neither class provided the most efficient way to burn calories. But I've explained why that aspect of the activity wasn't important to me. I simply wanted to send the message that physical activity is good. And this was a great way to do it. During those hours Bea was moving and enjoying it, and at least that time wasn't being spent eating.

CHAPTER 11

"You're up about half a pound," the third-string nutritionist lady noted pleasantly when Bea stepped on the scale.

"I don't know if that reading is really accurate," I interjected. "She usually wears leggings. Today she's wearing jeans."

"It's okay," the third-string nutritionist said. "Sometimes the scale goes up."

"Well, yes," I said defensively. "But in this case, I really do think it's the fact that she's wearing jeans."

Upon arriving at the nutrition doctor's office that March day, we'd been greeted by the nice but ineffectual third nutritionist. But she wasn't alone. There was yet another new woman sitting in with her, apparently learning the ropes. This was the fourth person Bea, David, and I had met in this office. Yet another person who didn't know us or our history but who was going to be privy to our weigh-ins and hear our personal details. For me, it wasn't a big deal. And David seemed to take it in stride. But Bea was visibly withdrawn.

As Bea had prepared to step on the scale, I'd noticed that she was wearing jeans. Not legging-type jeans: real, heavy denim jeans with buttons and a zipper and pockets. I knew right away this was going to affect what the scale said, and I encouraged her to take them off before weighing in. She refused. Understandably, she didn't want to take her pants off in a room full of people, including one near-stranger and one complete stranger.

In case you're wondering, I'll skip ahead a bit and tell you that I went home that night and got on the scale holding a pair of Bea's leggings, then got on a second time holding the jeans. Yes, I really did this. And guess what? I was a pound heavier with the jeans. So my concern that the jeans weighed more than the leggings was not unfounded.

The mood had turned sour from the discouraging weigh-in, although we'd arrived feeling positive. I was proud of our new exercise regimen. We'd made it through our Mexico vacation with admirable restraint, more or less keeping to our daily and weekly targets despite loads of temptation. To lighten the mood, I changed the subject.

"We just got back from Mexico!" I announced.

"How was it?" the third-string nutritionist asked.

"Great," I said. "Everyone was really awesome about staying on the program. Bea worked really hard and did a great job."

"It's okay. It can be really hard to eat right on vacation," she said, her voice dripping with understanding. My blood pressure started to rise. Why was this woman not getting it?

"She did great on vacation. She actually should be commended for how she did. I really think it's the jeans."

"How did you do on vacation, David?" she asked.

Silently Bea walked out of the room.

She went into the waiting room and started putting on her shoes. I waited a few seconds for the nutritionist to stop talking to David, whose vacation food choices were really kind of beside the point. I expected she would follow Bea to the waiting room to talk to her privately, or at least call out to her and ask what was wrong. But she did nothing of the sort. So I went out there.

I sat next to Bea, who was looking down at the floor.

I overheard the nutritionist continue the appointment with David. "Did you try any Mexican food?" she asked. I could not believe that conversation was going on while Bea had stormed out and no one had even blinked.

"Are you okay?" I asked Bea.

"No," she said.

"Are you mad?" I asked.

She nodded.

"I totally understand. Do you want to leave?" I asked.

"Yes," she said.

"Let's get out of here."

I went back into the office to fetch David.

"We're going to go," I announced. "I'll call the office about scheduling the next appointment." And we left.

I expected to receive a call from the main nutrition doctor over the next few days. Surely, I thought, the third-string nutritionist had told her that a patient had been upset enough to storm out of the office. Obviously, she would be concerned and would call to see how Bea was doing. No such call came.

"What should I do?" I asked Jeff.

"You shouldn't go back. That doctor is annoying," he pronounced in his typically blunt way, which I found so amusing and also clarifying. "You understand how to do the program, so do it. I don't think going to those stupid appointments is what's going to help Bea lose weight."

Indeed, it had been an ongoing challenge for me to drag the kids there: David got little out of it, and Bea had twice left feeling bad because of how an apparent (if illusory) weight gain had been handled. They were delighted by the prospect of not going to that office every Friday.

For me, it wasn't such an easy decision. I liked the program, and I even liked the nutrition doctor. And we were losing weight. I worried it was foolhardy to try to continue without the structure and guidance of a nutritionist's supervision. As with Weight Watchers, as with Alcoholics Anonymous, there was benefit in going to a meeting.

But Jeff's argument was legitimate: this was something we needed to be able to do on our own. The goal was to take over the reins and maintain a healthful way of eating without the supervision of a professional. Maybe that time had come.

We didn't go back.

CHAPTER 12

The goal of any behavioral change is to do something you can live with independently. With our formal ties to the nutrition doctor severed, I wanted to make sure we were eating in a way that was sustainable for the long term. I wanted to make the program our own. I felt suddenly empowered to make some adjustments.

One of my first executive resolutions was abolishing unlimited late-night fruit snacks. I didn't like how the requests were escalating later and later into the night, how I felt compelled to drag myself out of bed to wash and slice a piece of fruit because Bea had languidly called out from her room for an apple—something that was now happening two, three, four times a night.

I'd wrestled with the fruit ban. Fruit and vegetable snacks had always been "free," un-fraught, and it was nice to be able to be relaxed about one food group. But I decided some limits needed to be set; it seemed to me that the volume of our fruit intake could, in fact, set us back.

I was careful not to extend this limitation to other times of day. Between after-school snack and dinner, Bea regularly had three or more pieces of fruit, in addition to those she had at school, and I was fine with that rate of consumption. But I felt it was fair to "close the kitchen" at a certain point. I understood from talking to parents of normal-weight kids that they did it. So I figured I could, too.

Another area I felt needed work was Bea's relationship to food at school. From cafeteria fare to birthday cupcakes to class pizza parties, every day was a minefield. It was easy for Bea to feel isolated as the girl who couldn't eat what the other kids ate, but letting her partake without restriction seemed impossible.

There are millions of obese kids in the United States, but for whatever reason, we don't know any of them personally. I wish now that Bea and I could have looked just beyond our circle of friends—to the playground, the neighborhood, the buses and subways of New York—and seen that we were not alone. But at the time, all I could notice was that Bea's social group was comprised almost entirely of wiry children who ate whatever they wanted, or blithely left half their lunches uneaten due to lack of interest. There was no other kid Bea knew going through the same struggle.

I knew she had moments of feeling left out, because she told me so.

"I feel cut off from the other kids, because I feel like they don't have to go on a special diet," she told me. "They don't have to do something special. Just because I have to makes me different."

And while youth culture today wonderfully encourages kids to celebrate their differences, this particular issue is usually left off the acceptance agenda. I wanted desperately to minimize this feeling of being "cut off," as Bea put it. So I began by examining the behemoth of all school food: cafeteria lunch.

Anyone who's spent time in a school cafeteria knows the lunch line is not for the weight conscious. I get it—in the school setting, in addition to the expediency of not bothering to make things low-calorie, there's actually an argument to be made that lunches *should* contain lots and lots of calories. The school population is mostly made up of non-obese kids who are growing, need to be attentive in class, and probably run around a lot. On top of that, some of them come from low-income families that can't afford enough food. These kids need to get hefty amounts of calories for their lunch money.

Thus, far from having calorie maximums for school lunches, there are actually government-mandated calorie *minimums*. Which, you may be surprised to hear me say, is as I think it should be. The underweight, very active, or poor should not have to suffer smaller portions and fewer calories because Bea and others like her are overweight. When I buy a pair of pants, I know I'm going to have to get them shortened, because I'm petite, and pants are designed to accommodate the tallest potential customer. Once manufactured, pants can't be lengthened, but they can pretty easily be hemmed. I'm not thrilled about it, but I accept it. School lunch was similar: it was fair that Bea should have to adapt her behavior to a situation that was not calibrated for her specific nutritional needs.

I did feel that the calorie minimums were excessive, however, even for many healthy-weight kids. During that year, the USDA required that school lunches for grades K–3 contain at least 633 calories, and grades 4–12 needed to get at least 785 calories. And that didn't include the salad bar. It bears noting that subsequently, these minimums were reduced, and maximums were introduced for the first time, with New York adopting a minimum/maximum range of 550–650 calories. But I couldn't see how those numbers could ever line up with Bea's under-300-calorie lunch requirement.

Initial attempts to let Bea eat lunch like a normal kid had backfired just enough for me to be scared off school lunches for a while. When we first started the traffic light program, I had continued to allow Bea to partake in school lunch once a week, on "pizza Fridays." I didn't want her to feel alienated, and she had explained its appeal in such poetic terms that I felt it was important to let her keep enjoying it.

"Do you still want to have pizza at school on Fridays?" I'd asked her.

"Yes!" she'd responded. "The cheese kind of melts in your mouth and the tomato sauce kind of blends in with everything." When a food is described so adorably, how could I not try to oblige?

But fast-forward a couple of weeks to an early appointment with the nutrition doctor, when Bea had asked a question that alarmed me.

"So if I have pizza at school," she had asked the doctor, "can I also get something else? Like a cold corn salad?"

Thinking about this exchange now, I chuckle. A cold corn salad? That's my Bea. Not french fries, not an ice cream sandwich—a cold corn salad. She's so endearingly random. But at the time I was secretly rolling my eyes: *No, you may* not *have a cold corn salad. You're getting pizza, and you're trying to negotiate a side dish?* An insidious "salad," with its inevitable oil, lavished on corn, which banks over 130 calories per cup?

The nutrition doctor had fielded the query well. "No," she explained. "If you eat a slice of pizza for lunch, that has to be all you have."

But Bea's question confirmed for me that we were flirting with disaster by letting her get on that cafeteria line in the first place. Queuing up to snag her pizza confronted her with dozens of other choices, all of which had to be declined. Bea had been demonstrating amazing strength and resolve when provided with adequate guidance, but she still had the typical lapses in nutritional judgment that were appropriate to a seven-year-old. She wasn't ready for the responsibility yet. So I started sending her to school with a pre-made lunch on Fridays, and our experiment with pizza Friday abruptly ended.

Bea was fine with the shift. In the funny way that kids have of changing their minds from one staunchly held point of view to an opposing one, she had decided that school lunch was gross and that she preferred the lunch I made her.

Along with everyone else in the country, New York City's public schools are aware of the obesity epidemic and are responding to it. Education programs have debuted, gardening and planting projects have sprouted, and the cafeterias are instituting changes to make their offerings more healthful. Whole-wheat buns have replaced white, vegetarian chili has replaced beef, fresh fruits are available, a salad bar stands at the ready. It's a step in the right direction. And for the $1.50 I'm asked to pay, it's an unbeatable bargain.

I don't criticize the changes, because they may well improve the eating habits of some normal-weight children. While I couldn't imagine that Bea was going to be able to navigate the choices and stay within her limit of 300 calories for lunch (excluding fruits and vegetables), I wanted to at least investigate the options in the hope that one day they *could* be options for her. Even if the full meal being served totaled 700 calories, maybe I could advise her to have a half portion of the main dish and no sides, or a salad and a side dish but no main dish. I wanted her to have the chance to eat school lunch on occasion if it would help her feel "normal." I went online to see what the cafeteria was serving.

The New York City Department of Education's SchoolFood program provides calorie information to parents who are willing to go through the arcane recesses of the department's website to find it. I found the school lunch page via Google, selected the month and the borough I live in, and that month's menu downloaded to my computer. Granted, it was in a cryptic .ashx format with no further instructions on how to open it, but luckily I am a little bit computer-savvy, so I took a stab at changing the suffix to .pdf, and indeed, I was able to read the file.

The menu does not list calories, only the foods being served each day. To get the calories, I had to go back to the website, dig further to find the "menu nutrition information" link, and download that document. Once I'd opened it, I toggled back and forth between the two, looking up each item in that day's lunch menu and calculating the total calories.

It's worth noting that some of the items found on the lunch menu are missing entirely from the nutrition information index. And it would probably make lots of interested parents' lives easier if these numbers were printed on the menu itself. Just a suggestion.

My findings were not surprising, but not encouraging, either. A typical offering was Italian meatballs with tomato sauce, whole-grain pasta, toasted garlic rolls, and "Capri vegetables." If you leave out the available milk and other extras offered by the cafeteria, the nutrition info suggests that this totals about 450 calories. Another day, they offered mozzarella sticks with tomato sauce and a "Normandy vegetable blend vinaigrette," also coming out to about 450 calories. It turns out that most of the meals offered, from the hamburger deluxe to the chicken tenders, end up in the 350-to-450-calorie range, if you exclude the add-ons that bring the total to the USDA-mandated minimums.

Those are reasonable amounts for a normal-weight child to have for his lunch, given the recommended daily allowance of 1,600 calories for moderately active kids. But they were definitely too much for Bea. However, there was a new, seemingly better option on the horizon that offered hope that Bea could actually get back on the cafeteria line once in a while.

That year, Bea's and David's schools participated in a healthy lunch program under which the most nutritionally bereft ingredients provided by the DOE's SchoolFood program were jettisoned, and the rest were used to make more healthful meals. I knew they would be subject to the same USDA minimums as SchoolFood was, but I expected the individual dishes would be lower-calorie than their original versions. Maybe this new food would enable Bea to selectively construct a meal that stayed within her limitations.

The program's website boldly displays obesity factoids in a large font size ("We spend $147 billion annually on obesity related illnesses in the United States"; "In NYC, 1 in 5 kindergarteners is obese") and states that it seeks to "combat childhood obesity and to promote healthy eating."

The healthier lunches were already being served at Bea's school when David's school decided to introduce them. While often not available to attend PTA meetings because of work or family obligations, I made time to sit in at the one where the program was going to be presented. I was eager to get more info, since my thorough search of their website had provided loads of information but absolutely nothing in the way of calorie counts.

Let me be clear: I've never been That Mom. I don't show up at PTA meetings with a personal agenda. I am fortunate that my children attend excellent public schools with involved parent communities and effective administrations. I think the PTA does a great job, and while I suppose I'd speak up if I disagreed strenuously with something it was doing, I have thus far been content to stay out of it and let the PTA, the school administration, and the teachers do their jobs.

On the occasions on which I am able to attend a meeting, I'm usually both amused and annoyed by the parents who get up and rant about some aspect of what the PTA is doing, from how indoor recess is conducted on inclement-weather days to how much of the PTA's operating budget is being allocated to the chess program. These parents' issues generally have such a single-minded focus on the particular interests of their child that their digression is mostly a waste of everyone else's time.

But as I sat down for the meeting, I realized I *was* That Mom. And I understood her a little better. I felt a certain compassion for the parents in our mix who feel they must advocate for their kids' issues, even if no one else shares them—especially if no one else shares them. If they don't, who will? Sure, sometimes the particular flag they're waving seems marginal or even ridiculous. But it's true that a big-city school system isn't always set up to accommodate the needs of some minorities—such as overweight kids—and it falls to those kids' parents to stick up for them. Like with the Grinch, my small heart grew a few sizes that day in sympathy with overzealous moms at PTA meetings everywhere.

The healthy-lunch program representative stood up before the crowd of parents—none of whom, to my knowledge, actually struggled with an overweight child—and presented a bunch of grim New York City childhood obesity statistics before explaining how much better and more healthful the new program's food was.

When she was finished, I raised my hand, and she called on me.

I stood up. "What you're doing is great," I said. And I meant it. "My child actually has a weight problem, so I'd love for her to be able to eat this food. But I can't let her unless I know how many calories are in it. Can you provide that information?"

The lady was really nice, and so I felt a little bad, because I'd searched exhaustively for the information myself and was pretty sure that she wouldn't have the answer to my question. But at the same time, I was getting tired of people who didn't have overweight children telling me how to fight my child's obesity. So many pronouncements on how the problem should be addressed come from healthy-weight people with healthy-weight children. They tell us to make time to have dinner every night with our kids, to engage in regular physical activity as a family, to prepare healthful meals instead of relying on processed foods. As though these decisions were the reasons their children were healthy.

I didn't feel as if healthy food advocates were intentionally hiding anything about the contents of their meals—it just seemed like they felt the food was so unassailably wholesome and organic that it hadn't occurred to them that anyone would care how many calories were in it.

That's fine for the non-overweight kids. I accept that my child has special nutritional needs and doesn't have to be accounted for in every food initiative. But when you start invoking obesity statistics, you're talking about *my* child. You're giving me hope that you have a solution. So I'm going to need some evidence that what you're offering can actually help my kid.

If my child were diabetic, I wouldn't expect Department of Education food to adapt to his needs. But if a group preparing food for my child's school came in and told of the growing number of diabetic children in New York City schools and said they were there to serve that population, I'd be thrilled, and then want to see documentation of the actual sugar content of their meals. By the same token, if an organization is claiming to be fighting obesity, it seemed fair to ask them to back up that statement, not only with facts showing how bad things are, which are all too easy to come by, but also with data showing how they're addressing the problem.

The woman couldn't provide nutrition information for the food or tell me how to find it. Her reaction seemed to indicate that no one had ever asked this question before. She said she'd look into it. I never heard anything about it again.

With that one query, I outed myself to many total strangers in my community as the mother of an obese child. I felt it gave me special accreditation to speak on the topic. Like a black person opining about affirmative action or a lesbian speaking out about gay marriage. I was in it. My opinion should matter! So I became the mom with an agenda, an issue that was so specific to her child that discussing it seemed like a waste of everyone else's time. And I learned how little I mattered.

At Bea's school, healthy food offerings weren't limited to lunchtime. I started receiving emails explaining that chefs would be working with the kids to create healthful meals during class time. There was a day when they were going to make flatbread pizza, another when they'd cook vegetarian chili. Of course, the emails assured me, there would be no nut products, so nut-allergic kids could safely participate.

Parents of nut-allergic kids have a tremendous and stressful cross to bear, and I do not begrudge them any of the cautions they are afforded. A severely allergic child can indeed die from a nut. Many schools, including David's, do not make special accommodations for kids with nut allergies. Most restaurants, bakeries, food carts, and concession stands don't, either. It's up to the parents to protect their children as best they can when they aren't able to be there when the child is eating.

But there are a lot of other kids dealing with complicated dietary restrictions—kids with hypertension, vegetarians, kids who eat halal or kosher food, those who are gluten or lactose intolerant, and the overweight, to name just a few—whose parents also need to exercise vigilance to safeguard their children when they're inside school walls. Of course, an obese child's life is not immediately threatened by the presence of fattening, caloric food. However, obesity brings with it very real health problems—including mortality.

After receiving a few of the announcements about the in-class cooking series from the director of Bea's school, I replied to one of her emails. I asked her if the school could provide nutrition information for whatever it was the kids were making. I mentioned that it would also be helpful to know how many calories were in the new lunches served in the cafeteria, since this information had not been made available. I explained that there were many special days in which kids were invited to sample new menu items, and that I always had to ask Bea to sit out these occasions and stick to her bagged lunch from home. If I knew what was in the meals, I could maybe let her try them, like other kids could.

The director wrote back quickly. She assured me that she had forwarded my inquiry to the correct person, and an answer would be forthcoming.

That was the last I heard about it. So I tried a different tactic. I wrote to one of the parents on the committee overhauling the school food and nutrition programs. She was very nice and immediately responsive. She felt that the information I was seeking was probably of interest to many other parents, too, and she wrote to someone within the hierarchy of the healthy lunch program, seeking answers. No information came back.

Making my way through the bureaucracy of the school food system, I followed up directly with people from the organization coming into the schools to make the food. They said that nutrition information for the school lunches they prepared from the DOE's SchoolFood ingredients had to come from the SchoolFood program, and the DOE was unwilling or unable to provide it.

After several months and a dozen emails, I was finally deterred. I couldn't identify anyone who was responsible for providing nutritional information. So I gave up on working the system and took matters into my own hands, looking up nutrition information for everything on their menu using online calorie databases. Comparing those results with the original DOE's SchoolFood menu revealed that while the new program's food is way more health-conscious (less frying, more whole grains, etc.), it provides no caloric improvement at all over the usual public school fare.

Take this tempting offering: "Chicken Sabroso, Spanish rice, baked ripe plantains, black bean and corn salad, salad bar, and assorted milk." First of all, we need to contend with what "Chicken Sabroso" really is. I love Mexican food and live in a culinary melting pot, and I've never heard of it. I trust it's delicious and nutritious, but I don't know what's in it, so I'm unable to guess at the calories.

Let's be generous and assume it's three ounces of totally plain grilled chicken. Not very *sabroso,* I know. Let's also assume that each meal includes a quarter cup of rice, a quarter of a baked plantain, and three ounces of black bean and corn salad. Tasty and healthful, and a definite nutritional improvement over regular school lunch. But it's over 400 calories, excluding milk and salad bar and any other extras.

Another day's offering was Rachael Ray's Yum-O Cheesy Mac & Trees, which banks over 500 calories per serving (again, information I have only because I found the recipe somewhere else online and added up each ingredient's calories). All the new-menu lunches I researched, from black bean and cheddar quesadillas to ham and cheese wraps, clock in at the 400- to 500-calorie range.

I know, I know—calories are not the be-all and end-all of healthy eating. But calorie reduction was at the core of the system we'd adopted to help Bea lose weight. And neither regular school lunches nor their healthful alternatives fit the bill.

I'm really okay with letting school lunch be something only normal-weight kids can eat. I'd just prefer obese kids to be left out of the justification for nutrition overhauls that don't necessarily reduce calories. Is it a worthy goal to offer more healthful lunches to healthy-weight kids? Absolutely. Is it a solution to childhood obesity? Not yet.

I had given it my best shot and just couldn't see a way for Bea to partake in school lunch. Which is not to say another parent in my position couldn't have approached the issue more effectively. I could have volunteered my time to spearhead a low-calorie lunch initiative. Or I could have worked closely with Bea to prepare her to make the very limited and specific choices that would have enabled her to eat from the school's lunch offerings every day. But those weren't the right choices for us. So I made her lunch every day. And she liked it.

CHAPTER 13

For overweight kids, the world is awash with temptations and threats. As Thomas Frieden, the director of the Centers for Disease Control and Prevention opined, "If you go with the flow in America today, you will end up overweight or obese, as two thirds of Americans do." Even if Bea avoided school lunch, she wasn't out of the woods. More challenges awaited.

At 9:30 a.m., a scant hour after they've arrived at school, the kids in Bea's class are trotted down to the cafeteria to eat the snacks they've all brought from home.

When we'd started the program, Bea got a green-light food as her morning snack. Along with a piece of fruit, I'd throw in a 100-calorie snack bag, or maybe some hummus and carrots. When I decided I had to cut back on the number of junky 100-calorie packs I was giving her every day, I split one serving between lunch and snack, instead of giving her a full one for each. Now I felt I needed to take it a step further.

I know that as a person loses weight, her newly smaller body requires fewer calories to maintain its size, so calories need to be reduced for weight loss to continue. I had expected that, as time went on, I might have to adjust Bea's food intake downward. Bea was losing less than half of the doctor-approved half pound per week. When we'd begun, the nutrition doctor had said that if weight loss stalled, we would reduce her daily calories. I felt like I had room to make some cuts. So I shifted her morning snack to be fruit only.

"Why was there only fruit in my snack today?" she asked the first day it happened.

I wondered how much to tell her about my seemingly whimsical decision. Should the snack just disappear "because Mommy said so," or should I explain the physical and metabolic changes she was experiencing and describe their impact on her rate of weight loss?

"I think fruit is a good snack by itself," I said. "This way, you can have a little treat as your afternoon snack."

This was a specious argument, because she had eaten a treat as her afternoon snack from day one, but for whatever reason, she didn't push back on it.

Part of why I felt confident unilaterally cutting out calories is that I felt like these missed treats were constantly being made up for in unexpected ways. On any given week of the thirty-six she's in school each year, one of Bea's twenty-four classmates was probably celebrating a birthday, which means it's cupcake time. The year after we started this regimen, Bea's teachers made the incredibly great decision to group kids' in-class birthday celebrations together. All kids in her grade with September birthdays would be feted on the same day, with one treat, one class interruption, and one singing of "Happy Birthday." It's a great idea. It saves time, parental inconvenience and expense, and thousands of calories every year. I was especially happy I hadn't had to be the one to suggest it or lobby for its adoption.

While I'd hoped the policy applied to the whole school, it unfortunately did not. When Bea reached fourth grade, the teachers had a different plan: Not only would each child's birthday be commemorated individually, but the kids would celebrate each one together as a grade, not as a class. So now there would be forty-eight opportunities for cupcakes, instead of the twelve we had to contend with the previous year. Forty-eight cupcakes at an average of 300 calories each (the count for a classic small vanilla cupcake at Crumbs Bake Shop) equals 14,400 calories a year. Unless kids account for those calories elsewhere through reduced eating or increased activity, each can expect to gain more than four pounds per year, just from school birthday observances.

But during the first year of our struggle, we contended with the birthday celebrations of just the twenty-four kids in Bea's class. Every time one came up, I was reminded of a parent orientation session I went to at a very progressive, arty preschool Bea attended for a year when she was three. The teachers and administrators were talking about policies for school birthday celebrations and how they wanted parents to bring in healthful, non-sugary, non-processed foods to commemorate birthdays.

One of the school's founders stood up and proclaimed, "Let's raise the bar on cupcakes." My husband and I thought it was the most twee thing we'd ever heard. But on Bea's birthday, I obligingly brought in a cornucopia of fruit plus bamboo skewers so the kids could thread their own kebabs, and they were perfectly happy. On other birthdays, kids celebrated with banana bread or zucchini muffins. No one rebelled or even complained. The norm shifted effortlessly, and every family along with it.

Which made me realize now: *That preschool founder guy was right!* Why should we be teaching kids that every celebration involves mainlining glucose? Why aren't we instead challenging them—and ourselves—to come up with a festive but more healthful alternative?

Along with birthdays, there are the myriad other in-school celebrations that inevitably involve food: holiday parties, end-of-the-year celebrations, pizza or ice cream handouts to reward the kids for some achievement. Even if the food at these occasions is well-balanced, which many parents see to it that it is, it still needs to be accounted for in Bea's diet.

Most of these school-initiated occasions are announced in advance, and so Bea and I could plan around them. When there was a Valentine's Day party, I correctly predicted that candy would be rampant, so I eliminated about 100 calories elsewhere and told Bea she could pick one piece of candy to eat.

When French Heritage Day came around, with its attendant croissants and brioches, I was informed via email. In addition to a brief Francophilic performance in the auditorium, the celebration would be focused on a parent-prepared buffet in the cafeteria at lunchtime. I'd intended to discuss it with Bea, strategize, and maybe tell her she could look at everything and pick one or two things to eat. But I forgot, and she went in unprepared.

When I picked her up from the school bus later that day, she reminded me that it was a special day: "Today was French Heritage Day."

Oh, God, I thought.

"What did you have at the buffet?" I asked, trying to keep my voice level.

The list began. "A small chocolate mousse . . ."

Okay . . .

" . . . two pieces of Brie on crackers . . ."

Here we go . . .

" . . . steak on a baguette—two pieces of that . . ."

Huh?

" . . . a mini quiche, and a breadstick. A small one."

Um . . .

"And that's it."

"Are you sure that's it?" I asked, my tone not betraying the irony I felt in asking.

"Oh, right: two little pieces of chocolate."

Got it.

Mind you, this was on top of the lunch and snack I had sent with her to school. By my calculations, the calorie count was near 800—half her day's intake!

"Did other kids eat that much?" I asked, genuinely curious. After insisting briefly that they had, she adjusted her estimate to confess that other kids probably only had between two and five samples, not nine or ten.

My mind raced as I tried to figure out how I could possibly salvage the situation. It was Friday, so our week's permitted red-light indulgences had long since been used up. Her French Heritage indiscretion had more than overdrawn the balance in her food account for the rest of the day.

She'd enjoyed the Gallic treats at about one o'clock, so I knew she'd get hungry. I had to come up with a plan. I decided she could eat a salad with nonfat dressing for dinner, with some fruit for dessert. I figured I'd throw in a little whipped cream with the fruit, just to show her I wasn't upset with her. I knew that wouldn't be a lot of food, and I explained to her that it wasn't her normal dinner, that she'd had a lot of extra food at school, so we were going to have a really light meal that night.

It was the most severe food-cutting move I'd ever considered, but I went ahead with it. I knew she had ingested more than enough food to make it through the rest of the day. A child who eats 700–800 extra calories at lunch is not going to starve to death if she does not get dinner. Even if she hadn't eaten all that extra food, she was hardly going to suffer malnutrition from skipping one meal.

Bea's diet was, among other things, a test of her maturity and accountability. As we went along, I was figuring out what was reasonable to ask of her. She knew I let her get away with some deviation from the program and that ordinarily she could expect more guidance from me when confronting something as unexpected and calorically complicated as French Heritage Day. But she had a food budget and knew what it was. This had been an unplanned test of how she could handle such a situation, and it hadn't gone well. I wanted to make it into a teachable moment.

I think it served that purpose. When Spanish Heritage Day was observed many months later, I had learned enough to remember to discuss it with Bea in advance, and she had learned enough to stop after sampling two dishes.

"So? What'd you eat?" I asked that afternoon.

"A small taco and a couple of tortilla chips," she reported.

I gave her an approving high five. From our previous slip, progress had been made.

From a long-term perspective, my hope was that the rigor I was enforcing upon her would eventually become second-nature habits. At least for now, 500-calorie school lunches and in-class pizza parties aren't going anywhere. At this point, thanks to the positive nutritional changes many schools have made, the schools aren't doing such a bad job feeding our children. It was Bea who had to adapt, and it was my job to be her ever-vigilant ambassador and counsel.

The efforts I had to take to steer Bea through these obstacles were overwhelming. I was no supermom. I hadn't signed up for this. But I was doing my best to rise to the challenge and not back down.

I was fascinated by what I had learned. I kept finding myself yammering to friends about the divide between healthy eating and weight-loss eating and how efforts to address the childhood obesity epidemic had it all wrong. People could talk all they wanted about organic foods, less computer time, and whole-grain whatever. But for an obese child, losing weight is not that easy. The cold, hard truth, it was now obvious to me, is that the Herculean task of helping an overweight child required, at the very least, an acknowledgment that the child has a weight problem, and a willingness to reduce his caloric intake. It was also crucial that someone—probably the kid's parent—worked his or her hardest to help that child on a strict and consistent basis.

To me, the national fear of telling overweight kids that they have a problem was a huge contributor in the obesity epidemic. And the even-bigger fear of introducing the idea of a diet to a child, of *actually feeding him less food,* was compounding the problem.

Until we were willing to acknowledge this disease and confront it head-on rather than dance around it and talk about "moving more" or "adding in more fruits and vegetables," I explained to anyone who would listen, nothing was going to change for these kids.

I felt I could help be an agent of this change. I was passionate about this issue, and as a loving yet no-nonsense parent of an obese child who was actually losing weight—who better to try to get the word out?

But I was preaching to agnostics. None of my friends had overweight kids. Now that Bea had successfully lost some weight, most of them agreed with my rants and applauded me for what I was doing. But no one in my circle was really going to benefit from what I had to say.

Then an idea came to me at work. Instead of my having to adapt the recipes in the TV cooking shows I worked on, to make them low-calorie enough for Bea, what if the show itself did that? A program for people with overweight kids that demonstrates how to make normal, family-friendly recipes that are actually low-calorie! No one was doing that! It'd be a really useful show. A crucially important one. A gold mine! So I brought the idea to my boss, a smart, experienced television producer who has three grown children of his own.

He listened to my pitch and gave me a verbal pat on the back for my enthusiasm and effort, but he passed. "As a producer, I would never make a show that used the word *diet* and *children* in the same breath," he said. "I just hate the stigma of the word and I don't want to pass it on to another generation. I don't use the words *fat* or *diet* in my house. When I was a kid, my mom's experience with different diets ingrained in me a belief that diets don't work."

The comments stung a little bit. I suddenly lost a bit of confidence in my insistence on owning those terms. For my family, I was defining *diet* as a long-term, ongoing adjustment to how we deal with food. But the rest of the world still saw diets as temporary, inevitably ineffective measures, with the lost weight invariably returning when the dieter resumed her normal habits. I believe that diets *do* work—you just can't ever go off them.

My boss further explained that he had already tried selling networks on similar ideas, to no avail. "It's a tough slog. TV wants sensationalism—it wants *Dance Moms* or *Toddlers and Tiaras,*" he said, invoking the names of two series that had gained notoriety (and huge ratings) that year for documenting the antics of dreadfully overbearing adults and their exploited children.

He did note that there were a few heavy hitters in the intersection of television and food who were already addressing this issue pretty effectively, such as Jamie Oliver and his Food Revolution, or Rachael Ray's Yum-O organization.

Of course, I'd heard about these chefs' efforts. I own the *Jamie's Food Revolution* cookbook, and I recognized Rachael Ray's Yum-O organization from the appearance of some of its meals on Bea's lunch menu. I've used both of their recipes when cooking for my family. But in every instance I've had to cut the serving sizes in half, leave out some of the called-for oil, or in some other way adapt the recipe to be not only nutritious—which is certainly is—but also lower-calorie.

After my discussion with the producer, I looked at these chefs' initiatives anew, to see whether I had misjudged them. I hadn't. Jamie's broccoli preparation has 100 calories per serving, and his carrot salad has 188. I wholeheartedly advocate for kids to eat more broccoli and carrots, and if a healthy-weight kid who is averse to eating those vegetables is willing to do so if they're tarted up with lots of added fat, great. But at those calorie levels, it doesn't make sense to recommend those particular preparations to obese kids. A dinner consisting of Jamie's chopped green salad followed by one piece of his barbecued chicken with a serving of potato wedges on the side comes to 540 calories—too much for Bea. For her purposes, I can cut everything in half, and it's perfect. And so I do.

Apparently no one wants to make a cookbook—much less air a television show—where the dinners for kids come in at 270 calories.

I appreciated my boss's candor, and I knew he believed that I was doing what I felt was right for Bea. But it was clear that he was uncomfortable with the idea of putting a child on a diet. Few people without an overweight child could really relate to the decisions Jeff and I had had to make. No one who wasn't in my shoes could quite understand why I refused to let Bea have a spontaneous treat with her friends or eat a salad after she'd finished dinner, or that I'd prefer she drink Diet Coke instead of organic orange juice. I understood, because I used to be like them.

CHAPTER 14

One winter day I picked up Bea from school so we could go visit a friend's new baby. As we walked down a cold, windy street to the subway, I asked Bea what she wanted for a snack.

Her big brown eyes widened hopefully as she looked up at me and asked for hot chocolate. I don't understand Bea's love for hot chocolate, being averse to hot beverages and the practice of drinking calories that might otherwise be chewed. But I understand that, for whatever reason, kids just love it. And on that frigid, gray afternoon, I wanted to say yes. I wanted to create a moment where the two of us could sit huddled together with Bea warming her mittened hands around a steaming cup of sweetness after a long day at school. We stopped in at the nearest Starbucks.

I knew the hot chocolate served at Starbucks wasn't going to be quite as diet friendly as the 50-calorie sugar-free packets I kept at home, but I hoped that I could control the portion size and get it down to under-100-calorie territory. I looked up at the calories posted on the menu as I ordered. The kids' hot chocolate was not listed as a discrete item. The menu read, *Kids' drinks: 120–210.* That span covered milk, apple juice, and hot chocolate and was not sufficient information. If the drink was 120 calories, I could pour out about half an inch of it and let Bea finish the rest. If it was 210, I had to make her stop halfway. It was actually a fairly significant span.

As the barista prepared Bea's drink, I flipped open one of the nutritional-information pamphlets positioned on the counter. Again, no specific calorie count was provided for the hot chocolate. Hm. According to the laws of the state of New York, this place was required to post the calorie content of its beverages. To my mind, they weren't doing such a hot job.

"Excuse me," I said as the barista placed the frothy, steaming cup of hot chocolate on the counter and I passed it along to Bea. "Can you tell me how many calories this has?" My tone was cordial, and I let Bea start sipping away before getting the information. But I had a feeling this wasn't going to be a satisfying exchange.

"Sure," he said, and looked up at the overhead menu I had first turned to for the information.

"It's not there," I said.

He grabbed one of the nutrition information pamphlets. "Not there, either," I said. "I checked already."

Bea blew into the small hole in the plastic lid of her drink, trying to cool it down, oblivious to my inquiries. Fortunately, there was no one else waiting to distract the barista from this task.

"Do you want me to check in the back?" he asked.

"Yes, please," I responded. "I know it's somewhere between a hundred and twenty and two hundred and ten, but it's kind of important for me to know."

He retreated through the swinging door behind him. Bea kept drinking. Minutes passed. Many sips of this beverage, with its mysterious calorie count, were consumed.

The barista returned. "I wasn't able to find it," he said. "I could check on the computer."

"Can you, please?" I said.

He went back behind the swinging door again. Bea continued drinking. I was starting to be late to visit my friend. With every passing minute, more of the hot chocolate was disappearing from the cup, and I didn't know at what cost.

Finally the guy came back out again. "Okay, so it's two hundred and forty calories." *What?* "It's two hundred ten for the hot chocolate and thirty for the whipped cream."

"What whipped cream?" I asked. "I didn't ask for whipped cream."

"It has whipped cream," he said.

I grabbed Bea's cup and pulled the lid off. There, floating on the surface, was a bobbing cloud of whipped cream.

"She can't have this," I said gloomily. I felt upset at the position I was now in because of this counterperson's careless assumption. Now I had to be the bad guy, because he had made an unauthorized addition to the drink we'd ordered.

I knew he thought I was crazy, getting tense over thirty calories' worth of whipped cream. Well, I rationalized, what if Bea had been lactose intolerant and he'd added milk to her tea? Why did I not have the same authority to get upset? For the umpteenth time, I felt as though the needs of overweight children—to know how many calories are in something, to not have extra fattening things added without their knowledge—never occurred to regular people.

I was frustrated, not that others didn't care, but that I somehow expected them to intuit our needs and address them. This was Starbucks, I'd ordered a hot chocolate; what did I expect?

I looked at the half-full cup in my hand, knowing I couldn't hand it back to her. Calorically speaking, her snack was over, though I was aware she wouldn't see it that way. I felt trapped. I tossed the remainder of the drink in the trash, and we left.

I hailed a cab to get to my friend's house, because we were now too late to take the subway. Unpleasant and familiar feelings of self-doubt came over me.

I turned to Bea, who hadn't said a word since we'd left Starbucks.

"I'm sorry." I said. "I know that guy was trying to help, but they should have that information. And he shouldn't have added whipped cream without asking me," I said.

"It's okay," she replied.

"I'm sorry you didn't get to finish your hot chocolate. Was it good?" I asked.

She got a dreamy look on her face and licked at the faint traces of whipped cream on her upper lip, and we laughed grimly.

The incident haunted me for days afterward. I didn't like how I'd acted. It wasn't right to sacrifice Bea's drink to teach a lesson to a barista I'd never see again. But should I have let her finish the hot chocolate? I really didn't know.

A few weeks after the Starbucks incident, Bea and I went to lunch with her dad on a day she had off, while David was in school. We met on the street near Jeff's office, in a vortex of food choices of varying levels of appropriateness for Bea. There were a half dozen delis, a McDonald's, a Chipotle.

My husband suggested Chipotle. I wish. I love their food, but while I was on Weight Watchers I had done a calculation of what my vegetarian burrito bowl amounted to, and the results weren't pretty. Given that I required guacamole and cheese to be happy with my bowl, I was looking at over 700 calories. Maybe if I split it in half? Not even.

Bea wanted McDonald's. Believe it or not, that would have been fine with me. We don't go to McDonald's very often, but every time we do, I am increasingly convinced of its viability as a diet-friendly destination. People trying to stick to a particular nutritional regimen need two things from their restaurants: options and information. McDonald's offers both.

Of course, McDonald's is famous for such offerings as the Angus Bacon & Cheese burger, with 790 calories, 39 grams of fat, and 86 percent of the U.S. Recommended Daily Intake of sodium. Or the 570-calorie chocolate shake. But if you ask me, people who vilify McDonald's efforts to make its offerings more nutritious are being unduly harsh. McDonald's hasn't supersized anything since 2004, and there are many items that can satisfy the calorie counter and the nutrient seeker alike. The four-piece Chicken McNuggets has only 190 calories. There's a 150-calorie fruit-and-lowfat-yogurt parfait. Happy Meals come with apple slices and scaled-down kid-size fries. There's an array of salads, and the nutritional content of every item they serve is readily displayed. We could do well in a place like that. But Jeff wasn't in the mood.

We finally settled upon a place that had just opened, whose tag line indicated its mission was "de-junking fast food." The concept was to build your own burger by selecting your desired patty (beef, lamb, egg, veggie, turkey, etc.), bun, and add-ons from a range of choices. The nutritional information for each item was published plainly on the menu, which was available on paper, and on iPad tablets throughout the seating area. How perfect for us!

We reviewed the choices carefully and negotiated the specifics of our order. The establishment, in all its health-consciousness, provided me with a receipt that displayed not only the name and cost of each food item we'd ordered, but also its calorie content. Kind of cool. Except that, as I examined it, I realized the numbers did not match up to what we'd seen on the menu. The bread, for instance, was forty calories more on my receipt.

I felt I was being given an opportunity to redress the ways I'd mishandled the calorie information incident at Starbucks. I was not going to serve Bea her lunch and then take it away from her as she was eating it upon discovering it contained more calories than I'd been led to believe. This time was going to be different.

I went back up to the counter and requested a reconciliation of the divergent numbers. The counterperson called over the manager, who phoned the chef in an effort to solve the mystery. When the chef didn't pick up, he dialed the restaurant's staff nutritionist. This all took quite some time, and our food came out before the calorie investigation was complete. I ditched half the bun on my plate and Bea's to compensate for any overage, and we ate. I don't even remember what the staff nutritionist's answer was. I'd worked around the problem with Bea in mind, instead of letting my frustration with the difficulty of getting accurate calorie counts ruin our experience. While I'm sure the staff at this place thought I was as crazy as the Starbucks guy did, I like to think they—and Bea—found me considerably more pleasant to deal with this time around.

But it was yet another reminder of what we're up against, even in places that, on the surface, appear to be on our side. Healthful, I had to keep reminding myself, does not equate with diet friendly. Even though the place was overstaffed with customer-service personnel and even had its own nutritionist, a question from someone who truly cared about calories couldn't be quickly answered.

Things were predictably worse at places that weren't so health-oriented. At the Mediterranean place my parents loved, I'd had my instructions that no oil be added to my vegetables ignored. At a local burger restaurant, my request that Bea's five-ounce kids' beef patty be reduced to a three-ounce kids' beef patty was flatly rejected. And frankly, restaurants can't adapt to every diner's needs, so it makes sense that they can't be receptive to my requests, which are so detailed as to make Meg Ryan's in *When Harry Met Sally* look flexible. It's really not the restaurants' job to adapt their portion sizes and recipes. It is mine.

I did it all the time for myself. When Jeff and I go out to eat, if we order the same thing, we're served identical plates of food. Of course the restaurant doesn't make an accommodation for the fact that he's twice my size and more active than I am. I wouldn't expect them to. It was fair that our family, and especially Bea and I, should have to adapt to the realities of a world that is not constructed around the needs of children with weight problems.

But when you ask the waiter to bring out only a half portion of pasta and wrap up the other half to go, and he says the kitchen won't do it, and then you ask to speak to the manager, and she says fulfilling that request is difficult because they're really busy but she'll try, and then the waiter hates you and the kitchen messes it up anyway and you have to send it back until they get it right, and in the meantime, everyone in your party has practically crawled under the table with mortification . . . well, sometimes that's what I went through to get Bea's dinner on the table.

Frustrated by these constant roadblocks, I complained to a writer friend over lunch. I explained how challenging it was to feel I didn't have a clear voice in these situations. I knew that each individual moment—getting upset about something as trivial-seeming as a few extra tablespoons of whipped cream, for example—made no sense to someone without an understanding of the big picture. I couldn't find a way to express what was at stake.

"You should write about it," my friend said.

"I know, right?" I replied, chuckling. But a moment later I realized she was serious, and she had a point. A book could serve as a way to explain to the world why I was doing what I was doing. I could help people to see what I was seeing, and maybe help them better understand what the world was like for overweight kids and their families. I could write about how I had thought we were all supposed to be on the same team in this anti-obesity effort, but that I'd been disappointed to find so many people willing to disregard, question, or judge the intentions of a regular mom trying to help her obese child.

A book could impart my experiences to other parents like me, and maybe even include my little low-calorie recipes and give advice on how to handle school celebrations and friends' birthday parties. I could let parents know that they can broach this topic with their children, with openness, honesty, and love. I wanted to give other families the confidence to do what I'd been made to feel so uncertain about doing: help an overweight child lose weight.

The book wasn't necessarily going to be explicitly prescriptive—I was obviously no nutrition expert, and what had worked for Bea wasn't necessarily going to work for anyone else—but it was certainly going to be exhortative. All parents take responsibility for their kids' health and instilling in them good eating habits. For parents of obese children, this duty is brought to a whole new level above and beyond what is typical and expected.

I didn't know what to call it. One night, Jeff suggested that perhaps the title should be as straightforward as I felt addressing the issue should be. He suggested, *"I Put My Kid on a Diet,"* and I added, *". . . And So Should You!"* Yes, after six months of helping my daughter lose weight with moderate success, I felt I was ready to share with the world my personal solution to childhood obesity. Maybe it was an attempt to subdue all my real-world uncertainty with the bluster of an absurdly omniscient book title. But the more I talked about it, the more excited I got.

My writer friend was encouraging. She called her book agent, who was intrigued. Through that lucky connection, I suddenly had the opportunity to prepare a proposal for an actual book that would encapsulate all I had learned and accomplished with Bea.

Of course, every story needs an ending. I was beginning to wonder whether ours would ever have one.

CHAPTER 15

When I first located the Centers for Disease Control's kids' BMI calculator online, Bea weighed just over eighty-eight pounds, which, according to the CDC, gave her a BMI of 22.1, putting her in the 97th percentile for her age. An important aspect of managing the program on our own is that in order to make progress, I needed a clearer, more concrete understanding of what the goal was. Numbers were going to have to come into the picture.

Bea looked healthier, but she was still technically considered obese. So where would the scale, as it were, tip? Assuming her height stayed constant, if by the end of the school year, four and a half months away, she lost eight pounds—a reasonable goal on all levels—what would that get us? According to the CDC, a 19.3 BMI, which was in the 92nd percentile, and a move from "obese" to "overweight."

Okay, not bad. So what if she grew an inch during that time?

That would bring her to a BMI of 18.6, which was in the 89th percentile, right in the middle of the "overweight" category.

I went on like this for a while, imagining potential future dates, weights, and heights. It was profoundly obvious that the nutrition doctor had been wise not to get us focused on numbers. You could go mad.

Bottom line: I wanted to know what Bea needed to weigh in order to enter the "healthy weight" category. To get an idea, I calculated what she would have to weigh at that day's height in order to be considered healthy by the CDC. The answer was seventy-three pounds.

Wow. It was exactly twenty pounds from her starting point of ninety-three pounds. I like round numbers when thinking about weight. But it was a lot more than I would have thought! Looking at her body at the start of the process, I had wondered whether ten pounds might do the trick. When she lost the first few and I couldn't really tell the difference, and the nutrition doctor had intimated we had a long road ahead, I considered that she might have to lose fifteen or so. I really hadn't thought that such a small person, who was hardly the fattest kid you could imagine, could be twenty pounds away from where she needed to be.

I must admit to being demoralized. After all we had gone through—cajoling, arguing, doubting, manipulating, feeling isolated and judged, spending so much time and money—we were only a quarter of the way there.

I knew time and growth were on our side, slowly and delicately prodding Bea's BMI in a better direction even without weight loss. I considered seventy-three pounds our new target. When we'd started the program, I had secretly hoped we could knock off enough pounds to have her at a healthy weight by the end of the school year. Now it was March, and it was clear that wasn't going to happen. But could I hope she could do it by the end of summer? Five months to lose fifteen pounds didn't seem reasonable. But what if she grew? I went back to the CDC BMI calculator.

The BMI calculator gave me an outlet for my anxiety and provided a navigational tool when I felt I had no road map. I wanted to have a concrete goal in mind, but I couldn't be the one to decide what that goal should be. I didn't want my own judgments about appearance and weight to influence that decision. I wanted no less an authority than the U.S. government to tell me what my daughter should weigh. Once I knew that, I could predict how long it would take to get there. Psychology experiments have demonstrated that a person's pain can be ameliorated somewhat, simply by knowing how long the discomfort will last. And that's how I felt as I typed in numbers to try to estimate how long it would take for Bea to reach seventy-three pounds.

I didn't tell Bea about this goal, but I had it in mind. It surprised me that a child, ostensibly growing every day, could eat so very much less than she usually did and still lose weight at such a glacial pace. I felt that we were up against this fierce opponent who was not going to be easily vanquished and who was more brutal than I had realized. I had to be kind to Bea while also being ruthless in my fight against her obesity. Any instance in which we let down our guard—allowing Bea to skip karate, have an extra cookie, or get half of a big bagel instead of one little one—was ceding ground to the enemy.

So I felt little compunction about the sternness with which I approached our new tradition of Saturday morning weigh-ins. I likened it to how my husband had to take his blood pressure regularly to monitor his hypertension. It was a medical necessity. I tried to be offhanded or even jovial about it, but as far as I was concerned,

Bea could not start her day until she had gone to the bathroom and was standing naked on that scale.

"I'm hungry!" she'd say when she awoke.

"Pee, take off your clothes, and weigh yourself first," I'd say cheerfully.

Sometimes it didn't go so smoothly.

"I want a bagel," she requested one Saturday morning.

"Pee, clothes off, weigh self," I sang.

"No!" she shouted.

"You can have the bagel. Just go to the bathroom and then weigh yourself. It takes one second."

"I don't want to."

"Well, I'm sorry, you have to," I said.

She relented, stomping onto the scale so hard I feared she'd break it.

I was super careful to be exceptionally upbeat and supportive no matter what the scale said. If it was down, I was celebratory, but in a low-key way.

"Down a quarter pound. Good job," I'd say, nudging her off the scale.

If the drop was significant, I might get a little more excited. "Wow! Eighty-six-point-eight! You were eighty-eight last week!" On those weeks, I gave credit for her patience during the weeks the scale hadn't moved. "See, you kept with it even though the scale didn't move for a few weeks. I'm proud that you didn't get discouraged."

If the scale didn't show any weight loss, I'd encourage her. "Same as last week. Cool. Let's keep at it."

It wasn't until the end of April that the scale registered a gain one week. She went from 84.0 to 84.8 pounds. The previous week had been one of those big one-pound-plus weight drops, so maybe her body was just rebounding a little. Or maybe she'd had some extra food during the week, or just eaten too much fruit the night before. But I tried to make her feel okay about it.

"It's fine, don't worry about it," I said casually.

If there was a clear reason for her weight to go up, I talked to her about it.

"I think that's because we had that big dinner at Grandma's house last night, and you're still digesting it," I once explained.

I felt it was useful for her to understand that overeating does indeed show up on the scale. She didn't have to feel bad that she went a bit overboard at Grandma's house—but she should be aware that it had some small effect on her weight.

We are lucky to have many things to celebrate in our lives, and I didn't want those moments to be spoiled by guilt. I took the time to explain that special occasions are a part of life, and food is a big part of most of them. Weight management experts often warn us to be cautious about the connection between food and festivity, and certainly between food and emotions. "Don't use food as a reward!" "Food shouldn't be a requirement for every celebration!" "Watch out for emotional eating when you're sad or bored or angry!" But I disagree. We have cake on our birthdays for a reason: it's fun to eat cake, and social to share it. Eating does provide some entertainment when I'm bored, and some relief when I'm upset. I'm okay with that as long it doesn't happen all the time. Emotions and occasions can sometimes drive eating, and I believe that if you're conscious of it and aware of the connection, it has a place in life.

I was more concerned with everyday carelessness. Other parents often gave me grief for being too strict with Bea at any particular moment when she was presented with a tempting food no-no. But anyone who has tried to diet halfway can attest that partial measures don't work.

"Can't she just have a small piece? Just to try it?" a parent once asked, holding a slice of pie aloft above Bea's plate after she'd eaten her dinner *and* had some dessert.

No.

"They're kids for such a short time," a classmate's mom said one day at the movie theater as I handed Bea a sad little bag of 100-calorie microwave popcorn and she gave her own child a big tub of the good stuff from the concession counter.

I can understand that viewpoint, but . . .

"It's a special occasion," others often declared, as an excuse for giving Bea a treat.

But special occasions aren't really all that rare. In fact, they happen all the time. Today alone, as I look at my calendar, I see that Bea will be celebrating this month's school birthdays at lunchtime, and had the privilege of enjoying a *petit déjeuner* with her French teacher this morning. And it's just a random weekday! Both are opportunities for extra calories, and they have to be compensated for at afternoon snack and dinner.

I police David's eating, too, just in different ways. For example, his favorite food at Chinese restaurants is moo shu vegetables, mainly because he likes the pancakes. He used to eat *just* the pancakes. He'd have five of them at least, sometimes seven or eight. And then he'd be so crippled with constipation the next day that he'd be wailing in pain and unable to move. So we forced him to add the vegetables and to eat only a few pancakes. That's just obvious parenting. No one feels weird when I tap his hand and say, "Hey! Enough pancakes!" or ask, "David, how many moo shus have you had?"

When the mother of a heavy child exercises control over that child's food intake, it's impossible not to read more into it than if the interaction occurred between a mom and a normal-weight child, whether it's "That mom is too permissive; that's why the kid is fat" or "Good thing she's intervening—that boy could stand to lose some weight" or "That poor kid, her mom is nagging her about food just because she's a little chubby." Everyone's personal associations, value judgments, and emotional responses to my limitations were always hanging over us.

The nutrition doctor had a rule that discussions of weight should be confidential and that food choices shouldn't be dictated to kids. Rather, in a private environment, we should be working together to plan what Bea ate. Which, in ideal situations, we would. But for overweight children, most situations are not ideal.

CHAPTER 16

"Even if I fit in and I'm not fatter than the rest of the kids, that's who I was: the fat girl," Bea told me tearily. "And that's who I'm always going to be. Even if I change, I'm always going to be known as that person."

She was responding to her changing appearance as her weight moved down slowly but surely through the spring. She was within ten pounds of the goal of seventy-three. When dressed in certain clothes, Bea could pass for a normal-weight kid. That was new.

People had started to notice the difference. A neighbor in the elevator exclaimed, "Look how thin you've become, Bea!" Parents of her classmates told me how great she looked. Even a seven-year-old friend, his mother told me, remarked that "Bea looks skinny." Another mother used the same word at a chess tournament to acknowledge Bea's transformation. I put aside my usual defensiveness about words such as *thin* and *skinny* and happily accepted that they were compliments in this case.

In every instance, I made sure that people understood that Bea had worked very hard to get healthier—giving her credit for the achievement, so it wasn't just chalked up to a growth spurt or something, but also shifting the compliment away from approbation for being thin, and more toward congratulations on having adopted healthier habits.

But Bea didn't welcome all this attention. To her, it was a reminder that she wasn't like everybody else. I was confident that her young friends would soon forget that she had been overweight until second grade. But to her, someone commenting on her weight was an inherent reminder of the fat girl she used to be, and of the struggle that continued to set her apart from the other kids. It was impossible for me to discern whether Bea's discomfort with the compliments she was getting were attributable to embarrassment at the reminder of her former self or just the awkwardness of attention to one's body at age seven.

Bea still had her belly—and when I cuddled her at night and in the morning, I still enjoyed squeezing and kissing it. I wanted to convey to her that I loved all of her, even as we were both working so hard to make her a little smaller.

It was a daunting challenge to impart to Bea the idea that my refusal to let her be an unhealthy weight was different from a desire to make her thin. I knew she probably didn't grasp the difference, especially since my weight was healthy, but that fact did not exempt me from being disappointed that I wasn't thin. While I tried to stop expressing negative feelings about my own body out loud, I also tried to make sure Bea knew I loved hers.

I was focused on Bea, but in dieting alongside her, I was losing weight consistently, too. It was gratifying to see that by regulating my eating for the sake of setting an example for Bea—not allowing myself a gargantuan muffin for breakfast or two PB&J sandwiches for dinner—I could actually sustain a lower weight more easily than I'd been able to previously.

And I had never, ever in my life eaten so nutritiously. I was averaging three apples a day. I was even eating salads, since my husband insisted on them, and they were "free." Protein was an everyday occurrence. I was making progress.

I celebrated the kids' achievements with gifts for certain weight milestones. David got a present when he finally—victoriously—stepped on the scale and saw it had passed the fifty-pound mark. He picked an electric pencil sharpener. And Bea and I periodically chose a certain number lower than her current weight and tied it to some item she wanted.

Associating achievement with a specific number on the scale was likely not a strategy a doctor would have approved of, especially since we tended to celebrate in such superficial, girly ways. But I'm unapologetic. It felt right. It would be great if Bea could be motivated to stick to her diet entirely by the promise of reduced risk of type 2 diabetes, but that's not reality.

I'm aware that some experts say that our "reward culture" is bad for kids. But Jeff and I—and 100 percent of all the other parents we know—have been rewarding our children for achieving goals and improving their behavior since they were babies. There were gifts (bribes?) for potty training, for not fighting, for suffering through flu shots, for remembering to dress themselves and brush their own teeth in the morning. And why not? To a large extent, our new way of eating was a difficult and often annoying form of behavior modification, and adhering to it seemed to merit incentives as well.

I suppose I could have insisted she choose a gift with some gravitas, something that related to her achievement: a kit for growing organic vegetables, an encyclopedia of the human body, a special reusable snack cooler. But she wanted clothes, so I got her clothes. A few strappy summer tops from the Gap. A white, flouncy flower-girl-type dress from Crewcuts. The latter was particularly sweet because it was a dress she had wanted but hadn't previously been able to fit into even at the largest size.

She often asked whether she could get a hair feather as her gift, and I said no. Not because I felt it sent the wrong message, but because I kind of irrationally hated those hair feathers. In the spring of that year, salons were gluing or clipping colorful, thin feathers into kids' hair all over the city. A few of Bea's classmates had them, and she really wanted one. She also wanted pierced ears. (She also really wanted braces—go figure.) Some things had to wait.

In many areas, I encourage my children to accept aspects of themselves that fall outside the norm. I celebrate David's choice of pink as his favorite color, even as his peers try to shame him out of it. I don't make my kids attend some extracurricular activity they're not interested in, just because "everyone else" is. I don't even like the word *normal*. But as far as Bea's weight was concerned, I yearned for her to be normal. In this case, there was a correlation between a medically healthy weight and a socially acceptable weight. Being normal in this area meant maximizing her opportunities in life.

I wanted Bea to love herself and her body. I wanted to find the perfect line between insisting she not be unhealthy and encouraging her to accept herself as she was once she was at a healthy point, even if it meant she was still heavier than most of her friends or the girls she saw on TV. I wanted her to be vigilant about her eating in order to not cross the border back into obesity, yet not be obsessed with food and her weight. I didn't know whether achieving that balance was possible.

CHAPTER 17

When the summer arrived, I started to get concerned about Bea's height.

Having not set foot in a doctor's office for many months, I measured Bea's height as best I could at home, standing her up against a wall and drawing a pencil mark at the top of her head, then measuring that. These readings were obviously not exact science, but even in their crudeness, there was no mistaking the fact that she was not taller than four foot six. The measurements never, no matter how I tried to stretch them, ever exceeded the height I remembered her being measured at back in January.

This worried me for two reasons. On the dumbest level, I was bothered by the fact that her BMI measurement was not being helped by the growth I had expected. All the hopeful projections I'd typed into the CDC BMI calculator, in which I'd guessed she'd grown an inch, three-quarters of an inch, even half an inch—were irrelevant. She was still four foot six. And whereas a goal weight of seventy-eight pounds rendered her healthy for her age at four feet seven inches, at four feet six inches she'd have to get down to seventy-five pounds.

Three pounds doesn't sound like a lot. To give you a sense of proportion, it's equal to an average-height woman (like me) having to lose four pounds, which I can do in around two weeks. But given the rate to which we'd slowed, I knew those three pounds were going to take a while. Bea was losing a pound a month at best.

More alarming was that my seven-year-old seemingly had not grown in seven months. I was haunted by the possibility that all this calorie restriction had somehow stunted her growth. All those moms who had tsk-tsked at me when I'd denied Bea additional food, saying, "Come on, she's still growing, let her eat"—maybe they were right! Was her diet responsible for her stagnant height during a year when she should have been sprouting a couple of inches?

Plus she wasn't even losing weight! What the hell? No growth all year, and barely any weight loss through her entire time at camp? Something was very wrong.

Yet it seemed like every person who saw Bea that summer commented on how tall she had become. I insisted they were wrong, assuring them that I had measured her. It must just be that she was slimmer than she used to be, so she appeared taller. But she most definitely was not taller.

I shared my concern with Jeff. He told me I was overreacting, but was it possible that I detected a flash of worry in his face? I considered taking Bea back to the nutrition doctor, or at least to her pediatrician. I looked online and confirmed that Bea's caloric intake was indeed sufficient to sustain normal development and growth. I felt a little better after that. But eventually I decided to ask a professional.

I sought the guidance of a family friend who is a physician. He smiled at my worry and assured me that it wasn't possible that I had delayed Bea's physical development. I was relieved, but I was still perturbed by the standstill she had reached in both her height and her weight loss.

The new season and warmer weather gave me high hopes for increased family outdoor activity. We started having a picnic dinner once a week on a blanket in Central Park, eating our usual food and then climbing rocks, visiting a playground, or just walking around for an hour.

Bea's playtime with friends migrated outside, and I encouraged her to spend as long as she wanted running around with them. When the ice-cream guy showed up, we chose the Sno-Cones, which we discovered have only thirty calories and no fat.

When Bea started summer camp in late June, she weighed just over eighty pounds, down thirteen pounds from where she'd begun. I still visited the CDC kids' BMI calculator periodically to try to figure out where she should end up. She was still overweight, but moving closer to the 85th percentile, under which her weight would qualify as healthy.

My latest calculations involved what I might expect her height and weight to be at the end of the summer. By then, I reasoned, she'd surely have grown an inch, so she'd be four feet seven inches. And if she weighed seventy-eight pounds, according to the CDC she would be at a healthy BMI. We were so, so close!

My focus on this particular number was irrational for many reasons. First, it's a fairly arbitrary quantitative point. Seventy-eight pounds, I'd be satisfied. Seventy-eight-point-two? No. And of course, that's pretty silly. Also, these categorical determinations were based on percentiles, which is to say, the relative position of Bea's BMI number to that of other children of the same sex and age in the United States. But weren't many other children in the United States overweight? It struck me as odd to base these distinctions on a percentile number that reflected a progressively worsening profile as American kids got fatter. I looked into the issue and learned that these categories had come under fairly recent review. In 1994, an "expert committee" had recommended cutoffs for BMI-for-age at the 85th percentile, which was designated as being "at risk for overweight," and at the 95th percentile, which was considered "overweight."

In 2007, another expert committee recommended retaining the cutoffs but renaming them "overweight" and "obese," respectively. They felt that "the term 'obese' more effectively conveys the seriousness, urgency, and medical nature of this concern than does the term 'overweight,' thereby reinforcing the importance of taking immediate action." So the CDC was indeed keeping up with the times.

Unlike adult BMI percentiles, the kids' percentiles take age into consideration. I found the strict classifications to be a handy anchor in turbulent waters. But they could also get a bit maddening. For example, a four-foot-six, seventy-eight-pound child who is eight years and five months old is considered overweight. But a child who is the identical height and weight but eight years and *six* months old is considered to be at a healthy weight.

I had to set the goal somewhere. The borderline of healthy weight was as high as I was willing to go. I couldn't possibly go through all this and still have a government website tell me Bea was "overweight." I had to stick to the number as unyieldingly as I stuck to our daily food budgets and our weekly weigh-ins; otherwise, I feared, we'd never make it.

So the goal was seventy-eight pounds. With six weeks of day camp ahead, during which Bea would be running around in the playground every day, swimming once a week with her camp group and then a second time in a lesson I arranged for her, I was confident we'd get rid of those two pounds with no problem.

Unlike the previous summer, Bea's camp that year was a bring-your-own lunch affair, so I didn't have to worry about her overeating in a cafeteria situation. The camp provided two snacks per day—graham crackers, apple juice, fruit. After a bit of a snag in the beginning, navigating the right combination of these, Bea got the hang of it (water, not juice; fruit at both snacks, graham crackers at only one). Occasionally I'd come to pick her up and find they'd surprised the kids with Italian ices or some other frozen treat, but I tried to be cool about it. It was the summer, after all.

Bea was far more active than she was during the winter. She swam, she kept up her karate, she climbed the jungle gym. Her weight went down, but sluggishly. Despite all the exercise and disciplined eating, when her time at camp ended, she weighed seventy-nine pounds. She'd broken the eighty-pound mark, but it was not exactly the triumphant weight loss I'd hoped the summer would bring.

I looked back on all my decades of obsessive weight-monitoring and realized I had no explanation for what was happening with Bea. I'd previously considered myself something of an expert on weight loss (intellectually, if not in practice). But Bea had shown me how very little I knew.

My anxiety spilled over into how I approached Bea's occasional blips of overeating. At the end of her summer program, she and her fellow campers put on a performance of *Aladdin*. On that day, all the kids stayed on after camp and had dinner there before the show started. The counselor had emailed the parents to let us know there would be pizza served. As usual, I told Bea that she could have one slice.

The show was terrific. Bea was adorable and full of stage presence, lighting up her scenes in a glittering Arabian robe with a comically oversized, puffy hat. Afterward I congratulated her on a great job. I hugged her and told her what my favorite parts had been. I complimented her costume, which she'd helped make. I marveled at how much they'd managed to do in only a few weeks. Later that evening as I lay in her bed with her, I asked how much pizza she had eaten for dinner.

"One slice," she said, staring at the ceiling.

"Just one? Not one and a half? Maybe one and a bite?" I asked playfully. Still no eye contact.

Her little fingers started rising, one by one, to indicate how many slices of pizza she had actually eaten. Three fingers ended up in the air. *Three.* As it happens, I had seen the pizza they ate: *mammoth* slices.

Jeff was in the room, but I knew he wouldn't relate to the frustration I felt at the sight of those fingers. He would shrug it off, maybe make a joke of it to Bea—and believe me, I'm grateful to have a spouse who can find humor in these things, so there weren't two of us flying off the handle every time something didn't go according to my meticulous plans. But Bea's overeating by a factor of three made me feel like I was pushing this boulder up a hill by myself. It made me question why I was even bothering, and whether she was even on board.

We continued chatting about various and sundry topics, but I kept coming back to the pizza.

Were they half slices or full-size slices? . . . Medium-size ones? I saw them, and they weren't medium-size. They looked pretty giant to me.

It's not like there was a cake, and you had a piece of cake and it was like a special occasion. Pizza happens a lot. And you just can't be eating three slices of it.

Do you just want to give up this whole program? Do you even care?

I don't know what the best strategy would have been in this situation. Admittedly, nagging was not it. But I was stressed and tired.

Then camp was over and Bea was taking a nine-day trip with her father and brother to visit her grandmother, who was spending the summer abroad. I was staying home to work. For the first time I was not going to be able to steer any of her meals or snacks, or make any of the dozens of spur-of-the-moment food decisions that pop up in any given week. Only Jeff, who wasn't the ideal steward of Bea's diet, and her doting grandmother, who was prone to spoiling the kids with food as grandparents tend to do, would be in charge.

I was freaking out.

CHAPTER 18

While I had previously considered myself a pretty low-key, low-maintenance daughter-in-law, my communications with my mother-in-law in anticipation of Bea's trip abroad fell just short of frantic. Fortunately, my mother-in-law happens to be a dramatic personality and a florid email writer herself, and she apparently didn't bat an eye upon receiving my reminders, requests, and recommendations.

I sent a list of necessary grocery items (skim milk, cereal, chicken breasts, cucumbers, low-calorie bread, turkey slices, fruit, fruit, fruit, fruit). I indicated what Bea could eat for each meal and snack, including calorie ranges and sample meals. I warned about potential pitfalls (if all they had was regular bread, Bea could have just one slice—the two-slice option was only if the bread was reduced-calorie; corn and potatoes did not count as "free" vegetables) and generally pleaded for all the adults to make Bea's eating a priority so Bea wouldn't have to fend for herself.

My mother-in-law was totally on my side. "I will be careful," she told me over the phone. "I will do what you tell me." Once they were gone, I found that Jeff totally stepped up to the challenge. When we spoke on the phone, in addition to telling me about the fun activities they'd done, he'd give me a blow-by-blow account of what they'd fed her, and it was generally on target. There was usually something slightly off, one little thing wrong—for instance, the lunch might be about 100 calories over what was ideal, he'd give her a morning snack that wasn't just fruit, or there were a few bonus bites of dessert after dinner. But it sounded like things were going well. I was impressed and relieved that, in my absence, Jeff was taking the reins, even if he wasn't doing it as exactingly as I would have.

The morning after they returned home, Bea got on the scale. She had gained 1.2 pounds.

Now, 1.2 pounds may sound like nothing to the average person. My weight can go up more than that just from eating a big dinner. But for Bea, who had been working so hard to chisel away at each pound, and for me, who wanted to see her cross a finish line that would remove her from the medical category of morbidity, it was depressing.

I made light of it. "Okay, well, you just got back from a big trip, no big deal."

But I was confused. By all accounts, she had eaten carefully on this trip. Jeff had seemingly supervised her admirably. But my transfer of responsibility had resulted in backsliding.

I feared the moral of the story: that unless I was personally around to nitpickingly police things, this was going to be what we could expect. But I couldn't control things for Bea's whole life. I was going to need to let go. Like all parents, I wanted to place my trust in her at some point and let her take responsibility for herself. But this experience eroded my confidence.

The fact that her weight was back over eighty pounds made the relapse especially bitter. True, this was a completely arbitrary milestone—and 80.2 on my scale at home might very well be 78.8 on another scale—but it felt like a big step backward. My recent realization that she hadn't grown above four feet six inches had pushed the hopes of accomplishing our goal further out of reach. To go from a weight in the seventies back to one in the eighties was even more dispiriting.

And it remained so for six more weeks, because that's how long it took for her to get back down below eighty pounds. Six weeks! It would be October before we saw the other side of that number again. Those weeks were some of the hardest for all of us. I wanted to attribute the lull to the fact that she was finally growing, but I could see clearly, and feel quite palpably when I held her, that the belly I so loved was not getting any smaller.

I tried chalking it up to a weight-loss plateau. But this wasn't my first time at this particular rodeo. I knew plateaus, and this one seemed too long, too intransigent. I began to doubt whether I was equipped to surmount this latest stumbling block. I felt my capacity to guide Bea was faltering, and my energy was sapped. This battle, with all its required attention to minutiae and carefully calibrated emotional supportiveness, was hard for me to sustain.

In my mind, I pushed back the timeline for achieving our goal to just after Bea's eighth birthday. At that time, post-Thanksgiving but pre-Christmas, she would be going to the pediatrician's office for her annual checkup, one year after I'd committed to getting help with her weight. It would be a nice anniversary on which to reach the healthy-weight milestone.

I went back to my old friend, the CDC BMI calculator, conservatively estimating that she'd be four feet six and a half inches tall at the time of her mid-December checkup, an annual growth of only half an inch. At that point, if she weighed seventy-seven pounds, she'd be a healthy weight. At seventy-eight, she'd still register as overweight. So seventy-seven became the new goal.

But we were all a bit fatigued, and it started to affect how we treated each other when food was involved. Jeff might walk in the door with Pinkberry frozen yogurt some nights, and if Bea was up late, all three of us would dig in while David slept.

"Why are we eating this?" I asked him grouchily on one such occasion, as I dipped my spoon in for another bite, battling Bea's spoon for access.

"I think cheating is a fundamental part of dieting," he explained. "It shouldn't be eliminated from life."

Increasingly, during our weekly dinners out at a restaurant, Bea would get into a bad mood. Hungry and annoyed that the entire bill of fare wasn't available to her, she'd get irritable and say no to everything.

One night my parents took us out for dinner to someplace near their house, and I hadn't been able to view the menu online in advance. I looked over the choices and started running down the list of possible options for Bea.

"Shrimp cocktail?" I asked.

"No, thanks," Bea said wearily.

"Vegetable soup?"

"No, thanks."

"Mini tuna tacos?"

Head shake.

"Grilled chicken?"

"No, thank you."

"Share a burger with me?"

"Can I have my own burger?"

"No."

My mom, like many others, tends to proffer unsolicited opinions. At this tense juncture, she decided to jump in and suggest something on the menu I'd intentionally omitted: the salmon.

Salmon is totally overrated, if you ask me. It is one of those foods that are super healthy, which too many people have taken to mean diet friendly. It's not. Along with the yogurt and almonds I've already maligned, salmon is high in fat and calories, and in my opinion it's not particularly delicious unless slathered with a caloric sauce.

In case you don't know, a three-ounce portion of salmon has 156 calories and more than 6 grams of fat. By comparison, a three-ounce serving of top sirloin has 158 calories and more than 5 grams of fat. So go ahead and enjoy salmon's abundant health benefits. But I don't believe you're doing your weight any particular favors by eating salmon instead of eating steak.

For whatever reason, my mother seems not to remember my theory when scrutinizing a menu for things her granddaughter might want to eat.

"How about the salmon, Bea?" my mother suggested.

"Mom!" I replied sharply. "Can you not offer Bea something without asking me? If she wants the salmon, she has to share it with me, which she won't want to do. It has a lot of calories."

"I don't know about that. Every time I eat salmon, the next day the scale is lower," my mom assured me confidently.

"That's great, Mom. Bea can't have it unless she shares it with me." At which point Bea slumped lower in her chair and got a grimmer expression on her face.

"She is miserable on this diet," my mother muttered.

At that point Bea decided she would have nothing, thank you very much. To try to teach her a lesson, I said fine and didn't order anything for her. Then, five minutes later, she decided she was ravenous, and I had a Pyrrhic "I told you so" moment before agreeing to split my burger with her, which had kind of been my plan all along.

Once she had some food in her, she was her usual happy and cheerful self. But those minutes of low-blood-sugar consultation were unpleasant, and so was I.

Even in my grumpiness, I acknowledged that I was not totally without support. Many friends had encouraged my efforts. My older sister had coached my niece and nephew on sensitive snacking when they hung out with Bea, and she considered Bea's dietary needs when preparing food for family dinners. Bea's grandparents had tried their best to understand and follow instructions on how they should feed her when I wasn't around. Her teacher was understanding when I emailed her asking for specifics about what kind of food was going to be served at a school event. Some of Bea's friends' parents gamely played along when I asked if the kids could have only fruit for a snack.

Nonetheless, I knew not everyone approved of my mission or methods. I felt constantly defensive, anxious about other people's judgment, and concerned about how this whole thing was affecting Bea.

And while Bea was outstanding in her adherence to the program, the whining and complaining were repetitive and draining. We fought about some aspect of the regimen every day. In the meantime, I had to worry about toeing the tenuous line between being nurturing and tough, loving and strict, supportive and determined. And between packed lunches, David's separate dinner, and everyone's different breakfasts, I was preparing eight different meals and five snacks every day.

It was a lot. I started to criticize Jeff anytime he took the initiative to choose a restaurant, order food, or feed Bea.

If he ordered in food, I'd ask him what he'd ordered for Bea, then ask him to please call back and change it. The Japanese food order needed to be adjusted to excise the glaze from the sea bass and cancel the miso soup, which he had assumed was "free" but wasn't. Why was I the only person who ever thought about these things? When would I be able to let someone else dictate what Bea was going to eat? When would Bea be able to dictate what she was going to eat?

On such occasions, Jeff would often offer his irritated resignation:

"I'm done," he would say.

Done. He generally announced he was "done" when I reached a breaking point and expressed my stress through bitchiness. His ability to be "done," to walk off and leave me to carry on temporarily without him, underscored an essential difference in the roles we play as parents.

"Well, I *can't* be done," I responded at one point. "Someone has to do this."

That's part of being the heavy. You can never be "done." You can never throw up your hands. I hadn't undertaken this enterprise because of some philosophical idea; it was to help one of the three people I loved most in the world.

Jeff may not have approved of every choice I made in this process—God knows, I didn't, either. And as with every aspect of my parenting, there was plenty of room for improvement. But, damn it, I was doing *something.*

"You can't just be the martyr here," my husband countered. "You need to let other people take on some of the responsibility.

It's not helping anyone if you're the only person carrying the burden. You can't do this alone."

Jeff was right—I couldn't do this alone. But I'd learned that I couldn't rely on others to provide the support necessary to keep Bea on track. That left only one person who could potentially accept the responsibility for managing Bea's diet: Bea herself.

CHAPTER 19

Approximately once an hour, every hour we were together, Bea could be expected to complain, "I'm hungry!" But what did that mean? There were many possibilities, and in my soul-searching on this topic I have considered all of them. It was, of course, possible that her stomach was really too empty. But given what I saw her eat and how quickly she claimed to want more, that seemed unlikely. I'd also read that sometimes hunger was actually thirst in disguise. Was she maybe just thirsty? I suggested water, but that recommendation never went over too well.

I wondered whether she was confusing a generalized desire for food with physical hunger. It's an error most people fall victim to, myself included. There's hunger and there's appetite. It can be hard to tell the difference.

Then there are the times when emotion drives appetite. Maybe she was bored, tired, or stressed, or maybe she needed some special attention from Mom. Maybe complaining of being hungry was a way to seek comfort. I've discussed the issue of emotional eating and its appropriateness. But I mentioned that I think it's important to acknowledge the connection, not to allow yourself to just think, "I want to eat," versus "I'm bored and I want to cook something" or "I'm stressed and I would like to relax with some soup." I wanted to cater to Bea's emotions when they needed tending—either with support or with soup—but it was hard to know the root cause of each individual proclamation of hunger. Especially because there were so many of them.

So desperate was I to get Bea's weight loss restarted that I tenuously began confronting an issue with her that I'd avoided, despite my willingness to smash taboos and my refusal to let any topic be off-limits: I started challenging the veracity of Bea's statements that she was hungry.

It had started with the endless requests for nighttime fruit snacks, which I'd curtailed. Then I started feeling irritated when a single request for fruit came too closely on the heels of a meal or snack. She'd have just finished a filling lunch, followed up by a piece of fruit (or two), and then she would ask for a strawberry-and-whipped-cream parfait or other snack.

For many months I'd gamely acquiesced to these requests. Now, with my nerves more frayed and my faith in the continuing success of the diet shaken, I wasn't quite so receptive. I began to find her endless requests for food insupportable, not to mention exasperating.

My kids are not above exaggerating or perhaps even inventing physical symptoms to get attention. On a stroll in our neighborhood, David might out of nowhere claim his leg hurts and he can't possibly walk. I'll fuss over him for a minute, and then he'll forget about it and run ahead when I tell him there's a package from Amazon waiting for him at home. Random-onset stomachaches and headaches come and go with suspicious convenience, especially when it's time to go to school. When they're actually suffering from illness, which is rare, both Bea and David are admirably stoic about it. But sometimes they will insist they're not feeling well or are in pain when I suspect they're really not.

I think I have a pretty good ability to detect when one of my children is actually sick or hurting and when he or she might be inventing an ailment in hopes of getting out of going on a boring school field trip. But one can never be sure. So it was with Bea's hunger. It strained credibility for her to claim to be as hungry as she was as often as she was. But I couldn't really say with complete certainty that she wasn't.

My first step was to ask her to really think about whether she was hungry.

"Lunch was an hour ago, and you just had a bowl of soup and a banana as a snack. Are you sure you're hungry right now?"

"I'm sure," she replied.

Instead of sighing and giving in, as I had done previously, I introduced a new and controversial concept: hunger appropriateness. I told her she might well be hungry, but she shouldn't be. She'd had enough to eat. She was going to eat again soon. Now was not an acceptable time to be hungry. If she was, indeed, truly physically hungry, perhaps it was best that we teach her body not to be hungry when she's had enough to eat.

Thus I'd refuse her the requested snack—even the heretofore permissible-at-any-time fresh fruit or vegetables—and tell her to have some water instead. She'd just have to wait until the next meal or snack which, I reminded her, was never that far away.

This is what throngs of well-meaning parents do for their children every day. "Don't eat that now," we might say. "You'll spoil your appetite!" Or "Save room for dinner."

But once again, the idea of hunger appropriateness seemed like a spiteful invention when I applied it to Bea. I went over and over it again in my head: Was I right to try to teach her new, more healthful habits, including the idea that one shouldn't just eat constantly throughout the day? She had demonstrated an inability to regulate her own food intake. Weren't limits in order? Or should a young, growing child have the right to need to be fed constantly, and should I adapt to that demand instead of fighting against it?

I'd remind myself for the umpteenth time that these questions are at the heart of the discomfort so many of us feel about how to approach overweight kids. On one hand, I want to give Bea a pass about her weight, let her be a kid. I don't want to overwhelm her with concern about her health, her body, or food at such a young age. I worry that doing so will have adverse long-term effects, making her insecure or obsessive or saddling her with lasting eating issues.

But on the other hand, childhood obesity is a clear and present danger—and not just nationally but in my own home. Whatever steps we as a nation—and I as a mother—may have taken previously to try to combat it have failed. My efforts had been misdirected, too gentle, too erratic, or too late. This is a problem that needs to be confronted forcefully, immediately. There's no room for partial measures. I wasn't trying to slim Bea down a few inches—I was treating a disease, potentially saving her from diabetes, hypertension, heart disease, even early death. When I told myself that, I'd feel better momentarily.

"It's not your fault," I was careful to assure Bea when we hit a rough patch. "You're doing great. It's me. I feel like I don't know what I'm doing." At that point, the idea of writing any sort of book on this issue seemed like a joke. I was grasping for solutions to a problem that was bigger than I could tackle alone; Bea's weight had flatlined, and I was clueless. At a loss, I decided we should return to the dreaded nutrition doctor. But Bea was saved by the scale. On October 1, her Saturday-morning weigh-in displayed a drop from the previous week's 80.0 pounds to 79.2. And the week after that, she was at 78.6!

It's impossible to know what jump-started the downward trajectory. Maybe it was the crackdown on abusing sanctioned snacks. Maybe Bea had been on some giant plateau that she finally broke through. Maybe it was very simply just how kids grow.

In any case, we were both happy to finally—finally!—see Bea's hard work rewarded with a lower number on that scale after so many weeks of sticking to a program that seemed fruitless. Things were making sense again. The feeling that we had control over the situation returned.

Bea's eighth birthday arrived at the end of November, and she was so close to seventy-seven pounds that we began to discuss how to celebrate when she finally reached a healthy weight. Predictably, she asked for the hair feather. I considered all the sacrifices Bea had made, the moments she'd suffered from feeling different from other kids. What the hell, it wasn't a tattoo—it was a temporary hair feather.

One day, as we passed by a cheesy salon on Broadway that was advertising feather hair extensions, I asked her if she wanted to go in. She hadn't yet reached the target weight we'd set, but she deserved a moment of recognition and celebration.

She chose a thin, dark green feather, and the stylist hot-glued it into her hair. It was kind of icky, but also not that noticeable. I hated it. Bea loved it.

CHAPTER 20

As the end of the year neared, Bea's weight stayed under 78 pounds. While it dipped as low as 77.2 in November, it never quite hit the magic 77.

There was certainly no failure in Bea being seventy-eight pounds instead of seventy-seven. But since we were in this and were on a roll, I wondered if we should stay on track until she was safely into "healthy weight" territory. Was I wimping out by letting her scrape the floor of the "overweight" category and declaring that was good enough? If we stopped and relaxed the regimen, wasn't the only place to go back up, into the unhealthy zone?

Or was I just being overly dogmatic? I'd established the numbers as my guide and authority, and I was scared to use anything else as a gauge of Bea's progress. I decided I would let her pediatrician decide the issue. It was primarily her directive that had prompted this effort, after all.

I took Bea for her eighth-year checkup on December 21, and,

of course, the first thing the nurse did was take her height and weight. Right away I saw a problem. There was a new scale in the office. The familiar and seemingly irrefutably reliable metal Detecto scale with its double row of sliding weights (gravitas embodied!) was gone, and in its place was a slick digital scale. Rationally I knew that there were probably good reasons for the change, but I was not happy.

A digital scale seemed as likely to provide an accurate weight as my microwave oven's clock was of displaying the correct time. I'm sure it would be close, but it could easily be off by a half pound or so, and no one would know. I'm not sure why I felt like those Detecto scales were so rock solid, but it was what the pediatrician had used to conclude that Bea needed to lose weight and it was what I'd always seen in my own doctor's offices. A digital scale was fine for home, even for the nutrition doctor's office. But at the pediatrician's, I expected something with a little more authority than this newfangled device. My willingness to declare our mission accomplished now pivoted on what numbers would appear momentarily on its silvery screen.

Bea stepped on the scale, and I had a moment of reflection. I recalled the previous year's weigh-in at ninety-three pounds. I remembered the worry over whether I could help her, of my determination to help her, of the effort of helping her, of the frustrations and triumphs and surprises and disappointments. All, it seemed, leading up to this moment.

The digital scale displayed her weight as . . . seventy-seven pounds.

There it was. The magic number we'd been working toward, finally appearing on the scale. Granted, I immediately distrusted it, because it was a chunk lower than what she'd weighed at home just days earlier (and less than she would weigh when I next put her on the scale at home days later). But this was the pediatrician's office. That gave the number superior authority. The number 77 was being inscribed on her permanent health record, along with her height, which was . . .

"Four feet six inches," the nurse chirped.

If this were a scene in a movie, the mother would nod distractedly and then the information would sink in and you'd hear a loud screeching noise as her head whipped back to confront the nurse. Four feet six inches? That was the same height she had been eleven months ago, when we'd first visited the nutrition doctor's office.

Um, yeah, about that . . . It turned out that I'd misread the measurement of Bea's height that first day in the nutrition doctor's office. Her height then had been 52.6 inches, or 4 feet 4.6 inches, not 4 feet 6 inches. As a result of this inch-and-a-half discrepancy, all my concerns that Bea's height hadn't budged that year had been unfounded. She had grown nearly two inches!

The nurse was slightly perplexed. "Did she lose weight?" she asked, considering that a clerical error might have caused the unexpected decline in number.

"Yup," I answered. Proud, I smiled and winked at Bea, who sat on the examining table. She smiled back.

"That's great, good for you," she said to Bea. And then, to me, "If she stays at this weight, even if she goes up a little bit this year, she'll be in good shape."

The pediatrician came in. I was eager for her approval. It would be gratifying to have the same authority figure who'd prompted us to action a year earlier and who knew our long history with this issue confirm we'd done a good job. I recalled the time back in high school when I'd lost weight at Weight Watchers and then gone back to the hair salon where the stylist had told me I'd gotten too heavy. Prompted by my mother, he acknowledged my transformation. And that had felt good.

But hearing the pediatrician tell me Bea had reached a healthy number was even sweeter. "She lost weight, that's great," she said as breezily as she'd declared Bea's weight problematic the year before. "She doesn't need to lose any more."

"Are you sure?" I asked. "She's not technically at a healthy weight yet, according to the chart. I'm worried about stopping too soon."

"She doesn't need to lose any more," she assured me.

There it was: the final word. As a mother, you can't ask for a better endorsement than that. We'd done it. Mission accomplished.

Or was it?

I hadn't known how Bea would respond to the momentous occasion of her successful weigh-in. I considered the possibility that she wouldn't care that much. She'd gotten what she'd wanted out of the weight-loss process: she was no longer heavy, had eating habits we could all agree on, and had a hair feather. Still, I guess I'd hoped she'd take a moment to mark the official recognition of her accomplishment by her pediatrician.

When our appointment ended, Bea got dressed and we stepped outside of the office. I looked at her, beaming expectantly as we walked down the street. But she said nothing.

It occurred to me I'd experienced something similar before. I realize that breast cancer is not the most apt comparison to obesity, but when a friend of mine afflicted with the disease sought treatment and was declared cancer free, I had said the wrong thing.

As soon as I saw her, I'd given her a giant hug. "Congratulations!" I squealed.

But I could tell that wasn't the right thing to say.

"What?" I asked, backing off. "You're not feeling celebratory?"

She explained her feelings indelibly. "You know, people want to feel like, 'Oh, boy, now we can really put that behind us and move on,' when instead it feels more like my relationship with life has fundamentally changed and there is now a level of anxiety and loss that will be with me forever," she said.

She said that being happy didn't feel right. "I am a different person because of this experience. I have a new understanding about my fragility."

I thought of her words now, when walking with Bea. She, too, was different because of what she'd gone through. She was less carefree, more responsible, more knowing, perhaps even more aware of her fragility. She didn't possess the feeling of invincibility about her health that most other kids her age had.

"How do you feel about all the weight you lost?" I asked her when we got home.

"Good," she said, blandly.

"Do you like the way you look now?" I asked.

"Yes," she said definitively.

"Do you feel different?"

"No. That's still me," she said. "I'm not a different person just because I lost sixteen pounds."

The tone had become unexpectedly heavy. I felt a small pit in my stomach. I pulled her onto my lap and pressed my cheek against hers.

She went on. "I'm not comfortable with saying, 'Oh, yeah, I've changed everything and everything's going to be perfect for the rest of humanity,' " she said. "I think I've changed half of the way, but not that I fixed my entire life. Because that isn't true. Who can fix their entire life when they're eight?"

"Well, no, of course you haven't changed your whole life. But you're not overweight anymore. You did fix that. That part of you is in the past."

Her body tensed in my arms. She began to tear up.

"Just because it's in the past doesn't mean it didn't happen," she said.

Like my friend with the cancer diagnosis, the outcome of Bea's diet was, to her, not a victory, or even really an ending. She understood, even though I hadn't, that it was glib and reductive to act like her experience was one worthy of glee. Her maturity in realizing this, and her intelligence in articulating it, filled me with pride and sadness in equal measure.

If I wondered why Bea couldn't revel in her success, I needed only to look at myself. No matter how well I controlled my eating, I still had feelings of fear and guilt around food. No matter how many pounds I lost, another diet was just around the corner. Regardless of how far I had come since my younger years of obsessive dieting and negative self-image, I still had a complicated relationship to my body. And even if my eating and weight issues had evened out as I got older, I had spent many years being victimized by them, and I knew that was a tragic waste of energy, time, and self-esteem.

I am not an alcoholic, but I feel like I understand the mind-set of a sober alcoholic. You are managing your disease and have it under control at that moment. But it's still there in you. You think differently than nonalcoholics do, and you need to monitor your environment and your decisions differently. You must manage your behavior more stringently than someone who does not share your addiction. It will always be a part of who you are. There are similarities with being overweight. You can manage your weight, control your eating, even become thin, but that tendency is still inside you.

I had believed that I could set Bea on a different track, that I could "cure" her of being overweight by changing her eating habits before her self-image dimmed so much that she came to think of herself as a fat person. But I was too late. Or maybe it was never possible. She had indeed changed her body and her lifestyle, but the metamorphosis was bittersweet, because it had cost her some of the innocence of her childhood.

Who Bea was—who I was—hadn't essentially changed. There's no way for food-focused people like me, my husband, and my daughter to walk through the city and *not* think instantly about stopping at the mini cupcake shop (or, in Jeff's case, the falafel truck). We can only try to control whether we allow ourselves to go there and, if we do, how many of those amazing little treats we pop into our mouths. Being able to exert that control is a huge step forward. But the essential challenge of our attitude toward food and our "normative discontent" with our bodies hasn't gone away; I can't imagine it ever will. Bea realized that without my having to tell her.

It felt strange, but maybe it's psychologically to be expected, that as we reached her weight loss goal, all these emotional issues were coming to the surface. Suddenly we were confronting feelings of sadness and insecurity that Bea had locked away as she did the work of taking the weight off. Having reached the finish line, we were both taking a moment to look back. Some of the pain and frustration of Bea's predicament as an overweight child was bubbling up.

Meanwhile, I felt as anxious as ever. The pediatrician had told me we could stop, but I'd spent the last year refusing to stop. It was hard to halt that momentum. Plus the conventional wisdom rang in my ears: losing weight is easy (though millions of people would beg to differ); it's keeping it off that's hard. We were about to enter a phase that promised to be every bit as challenging as the one we'd just completed. We were by no means done.

CHAPTER 21

A month into the New Year, I was eager to introduce a "new normal" around Bea's eating. In response to the pediatrician's approval of her weight, I felt the time had come to loosen the reins slightly.

Bea ate the exact same breakfast and lunch as she had before. Her post-breakfast morning snack was still only a piece of fruit, and her afternoon snack was still only 100 calories or fewer, in addition to fruit. Dinner was the same size as before, but I reintroduced olive oil to our salad dressings. I also started preparing vegetables with a little oil—our green beans might have a pat of light butter on them, and our beloved Brussels sprouts were roasted in olive oil again, instead of just blandly boiled.

On the weekends, if we passed a bakery, we might have a little cookie or mini cupcake, which previously I would have accounted for more carefully. If Bea wanted a bite of her dad's turkey burger or her brother's pasta, I didn't stop her. I let her skip karate two or three times.

The changes we made were tiny, but apparently they added up. Bea's weight started to climb. At the end of January she was at 78.8 pounds. A mere week later she weighed 79.8. That jump was so significant, I was sure it was some anomaly due to water weight, and I was prepared to write it off. But the following week, the scale hadn't moved. And a week later, she was up to 80.6. Another pound and a half gained in a month, for a total of three pounds regained.

A little weight gain was to be expected. But three pounds was worrying. And Bea had traversed the psychologically significant (to me, anyway) eighty-pound mark in the wrong direction yet again. I removed all the reintroduced oils, cut out extra snacks, and required full attendance at karate. We got the weight back down to just under eighty.

But three weeks later, she'd gained two more pounds. I found the pace and extent of the weight gain inexplicable and scary. Once again I considered the possibility that she was just growing. But the visible growth of her belly refuted that theory.

One night, after she'd eaten a lot of fruit, Bea observed her protruding stomach.

"I'm fat again," she said.

Those words hit me like a ton of bricks. My immediate response was panic that I had put that thought into her head. I knew that she had called herself fat many times before I'd put her on a diet. But this was the first time she'd used that word since she'd lost the weight.

It was particularly jarring to hear her self-rebuke on the heels of a period of weight gain. If she'd said it when she was at a more securely healthy number, I'd have chalked it up to attention seeking, perhaps even compliment fishing. But was she making a sincere self-assessment of her body, which indeed had migrated back, technically, into the "overweight" category? Had I created a situation in which, anytime she gains weight, she's going to think she's fat?

Either way, I refused to tolerate her talking that way. There was little sympathy in my response, because I didn't want to encourage her to use the word *fat* self-deprecatingly in expectation of my indulgently refuting her. I was firm. "You are not fat," I said. "You've just regained a little weight, and we're going to be more careful."

It seemed that the level of vigilance was going to have to be stricter than I'd hoped. But hadn't I been the one who wanted to return the word *diet* to its original meaning of a continual, habitual way of eating? Didn't I believe that the only way diets worked is if you never went off them? Why hadn't I realized that this was just the way it was going to be? We put in the effort, and brought the weight back down again.

We'd won a battle, but the war raged on. This diet wasn't over.

This realization that Bea's way of eating couldn't really change marked a major shift in my attitude. I didn't feel the same panic about reaching one particular goal. I accepted that we were in a pretty good place and that the process was ongoing. I didn't feel any time pressure. I became more relaxed about week-to-week ups and downs and occasional nutritional lapses. It was just life now. The focus of my efforts now had to be transferring responsibility for sustaining the habits from me to Bea.

I didn't get so stressed out in social situations or if we ate out somewhere. Partially it was because now that Bea was at a healthy weight, I could publicly discuss her food choices with her without incurring the judgments of people overhearing us. We were just a boring mom and a regular kid having a mundane conversation about nutrition. Finally we were normal.

Bea's weight stayed pretty stable, at or near the healthy mark. Limited as her daily menus seemed, they were necessary for maintaining her weight. It was not how she wanted to eat nor how her body naturally tended to eat. Which was all the more reason she had to eat this way. This was it. This was Bea's lifestyle now.

One of the most noticeable shifts was Bea's attitude toward her body. That measure of our work had shown great improvement. She carried herself with pride and even a little extra kick in her step. She dressed up for a party or donned a bathing suit without hesitation.

I began to feel good about what we were doing—and even my role in it. It occurred to me that maybe I could help other moms in my situation. I knew how universal this quagmire was, how uniquely helpless parents feel when they see themselves as having to choose between denying a child the joys of childhood or letting them barrel toward bad health. I still felt that for me to write an instructive book for moms of overweight kids, with weight-loss tips and family-friendly recipes, was ludicrous. I was no expert; the missteps, fumbles, and frustrations of the past many months had demonstrated that quite clearly. But I could tell my story and share Bea's experience, and maybe our personal narrative of what we'd gone through could be as inspiring as the guidebook I was not competent to write.

As my friend's book agent helped me adapt my proposal from a how-to book to a memoir, he also shared the thrust of my story with an editor at *Vogue*. And just like that, the editor suggested I write a piece for the magazine. *Vogue* was interested in what it was like to undertake a weight-loss effort for an obese child when doing so proved so unexpectedly controversial—including the embarrassing and low moments that illustrated how hard the process was and how challenged I had been.

I was thrilled by the opportunity to get my story out in front of such a large national audience of women. I had never written an article for a magazine before, but even in my inexperience, I was aware of the considerable irony in writing about weight in a magazine that glorifies an unhealthy standard of female thinness. But it made a perverse kind of sense to me: maybe *Vogue* was just the right forum in which to write about how women like me sometimes need to put aside their insecurities—which fashion magazines had played a role in solidifying—in order to help their own children with health-threatening weight problems.

My article was to be featured in the "Up Front" section, which may well be renamed "Upper-Class White People's Problems." Its contents generally consist of essays by well-to-do women about their tribulations. Sometimes it's something as serious as a chronic illness or the loss of a child. More often the articles center on romantic entanglements, spiritual quests, or luxurious efforts at self-improvement.

The problem I was writing about was not really one that affected rich people all that much. Overweight and obese Americans are disproportionately found in poorer populations. There's a statistical correlation between obesity and lower socioeconomic status. I wasn't sure whether *Vogue*'s readership would necessarily relate personally to my issue, but I felt the magazine provided a reputable, respectable forum in which to present it.

The column's lengthy, first-person format would allow me to tell our story and get this issue out in the open: how taking on Bea's weight problem made me the subject of unexpected judgment, hypocrisy, and isolation. How parents of obese kids fear damaging their children so much that they are paralyzed, unable to even broach the topic, leaving their children floundering. How schools, other parents, everyday food situations, and even healthful-eating initiatives inadvertently set obese children up to fail.

Vogue also wanted to photograph Bea and me together. When I shared that news with Bea, she was excited. But then one day she wasn't so sure.

"If you are not comfortable with this article, tell me, and I will not write it," I told Bea. "It is not a big deal at all. It is not worth it to write it if it will make you feel bad."

"No, I want you to. I just don't know if I want to be in the picture," she said.

Her concern shook me enough that I reconsidered the idea of writing the essay at all. I'd previously mulled the cons of immortalizing Bea's struggle in print but had convinced myself that they were outweighed by the pros of talking about this publicly in a way that confronted our hurdles and celebrated her resilience. People wrote about all kinds of issues with their children. Why should obesity be any different? Any recounting of our experience was only going to convey how incredible Bea was.

I thought that, as a society, we'd moved beyond blaming people for their clinical diagnoses. We no longer think of kids with learning disabilities as stupid. We don't think drug addiction is the result of weak will. Mental illness is not something we expect people to just "snap out of" or keep under control. These are diseases that require help and intervention. Yet there's still a powerful stigma attached to obesity, as though it is at least partially the fault of the lazy, gluttonous person who suffers from it. I wanted to help smash that myth. But not at the expense of Bea's feelings.

I called the editor and warned him that Bea was having second thoughts. I said I was open to the possibility that she might change her mind, but at this point we should prepare for the likely event that she would not want to be photographed. A father of two, he said he understood.

With the pressure off, Bea did an about-face and insisted she most definitely, positively wanted to stay in the picture.

I wasn't sure what to do. Jeff felt we should let Bea have the final say but thought we should seek a professional opinion. I called a trusted therapist who has extensive experience with children and always provides reassuring, sane advice when we're experiencing a challenging moment in our family. I explained the situation to him over the phone.

His response was quick and definitive. The magazine article must be written. And a book, too. The issue was an important one that nobody was talking about. It needed to be discussed, and given what Bea and I had gone through, I had a story to tell that was relevant and could be helpful to lots of other parents.

However, Bea should be left out of it, he said. She should not collaborate on the book, as I had considered. And she should not appear in the *Vogue* magazine photo. This was my work. Bea should be kept separate from it.

Good advice. Got it. Done.

"You're not going to be in the *Vogue* photo, Bea," I told her later. "I'm sorry I offered it as a possibility."

She was crestfallen. "But I want to!"

I was adamant. "Sorry, no."

Days went by, and Bea reminded me repeatedly that she really, really wanted to be in the photo. She said this was something we'd accomplished together and she wanted to be a part of it. Eventually my husband and I relented.

We should have stood firm. I should have listened to the therapist's advice. But I imagined the article coming out, next to a big picture of . . . just me? The story wasn't mine alone. Bea and I were a team. My article was not about the efforts of a mother, but the journey of a mother and a daughter. Leaving Bea out of the image felt wrong.

I also wanted to give Bea an opportunity to celebrate her accomplishment—something I felt she had not sufficiently done yet. I knew she would relish having her hair and makeup done, trying on dresses, and being photographed by a professional photographer. In the shallowest way, I wanted her to have a once-in-a-lifetime day where she could feel like a star.

I also wanted to send her a clear message: *You have accomplished something so unusual that a world-renowned magazine wants to spotlight you. You played the most important, active role in getting where you are today. Even though you're just a kid, you took responsibility for your health and made really difficult changes. You deserve recognition.*

I probably protest too much. Whatever excuses I might make in defense of my decision to let Bea pose for *Vogue* are irrelevant. In retrospect, it was not the right choice.

On the Sunday night before the Friday photo shoot, Bea and I lay in bed together, each of us with a laptop. She logged into the Twitter account she had set up months before and rarely used (in the same time frame, David had racked up seventy followers and had written more than 300 tweets). She decided to compose a message.

"Going to sleep. Stoked for Friday," she began. I glanced at her screen surreptitiously as she typed, curious to see how she was going to describe the photo shoot to her handful of followers. "On Friday I have something at school called a teach-and-tell which is like a show-and-tell but you teach the class about something."

The *Vogue* shoot didn't even register. Good for her for having solid priorities.

That Friday after school, a photographer and his assistant arrived and rearranged our furniture while a fashion assistant wheeled racks of clothes into Bea's tiny room. A makeup artist and a hairstylist laid out their tools on our dining table. Plastic black trunks filled with shoes took up the better part of our living room floor.

Bea looked insanely cute in everything they tried on her. I wasn't such an easy fit. Even the collective powers of *Vogue* were hard pressed to find attire that flattered my idiosyncratic build. But the editor managed to pull out a multicolored sheath that looked good, so we went with that. As someone whose wardrobe consists entirely of black and gray clothing, I felt like a rainbow had thrown up on me, but how can you argue with *Vogue*'s taste? I was just excited to be there.

Since everyone asks, I'll tell you: no, we didn't get to keep the clothes.

CHAPTER 22

All hell broke loose when the *Vogue* article came out. From the reaction in the blogosphere, you would have thought that I had maimed my daughter.

I'd assumed the piece would generate a little buzz on the mommy blogs and parent-oriented message boards online. I knew some aspects of what I'd written would be controversial, such as the very idea of putting a young child on a diet, or my occasional choice of lower-calorie processed foods over higher-calorie organic fare. I was truly interested to see what people had to say about it.

So the day the issue hit the newsstands, I logged into Urban-Baby, a popular parenting website with an extremely busy (and often venomous) message board. If anyone had an opinion about what I'd written—particularly a negative one—chances were good it would end up on UrbanBaby. The site's boards were the ones I had frequented in my earlier years of motherhood, when I'd post or search to allay anxiety about my children's mild ailments or school enrollments. The site could be immensely and immediately helpful.

It could also be petty and spiteful, its anonymity releasing moms from the social pressure and moral filter that usually curbed the frank expression of judgments about other people's parenting.

I steeled myself and poked around a bit but found nothing about my article. Hm. Maybe no one really cared.

But within a day or so, it became clear that people did care. A friend said her buddy at the *Today* show wanted to book me for an appearance. My mother called to let me know that someone from *Good Morning America* had phoned her at home, hoping to get in touch with me. An email from a staffer at *20/20* found its way to my husband's in-box at work. ABC News hand-delivered a letter to my apartment building.

It was somewhat exciting, very disconcerting, and utterly bizarre. While I thought that what I'd written was worth talking about, this response was unexpected. I look back on the flurry of activity with a bit of disbelief now. I hadn't imagined that anyone would ask me to speak publicly about this issue. Other than what I'd written in my article, I didn't know what to say. I was totally unprepared for the attention. As someone who watches a lot of TV, I knew that responding to media requests when not fully prepared to speak was a recipe for disaster. I did not return any of the calls.

The interest from these TV shows was but a mild harbinger of the brewing firestorm. And if the entirely polite and respectful overtures from this handful of producers freaked me out, you can imagine how thrown I was by the nature of the onslaught I was about to experience.

Mentions of my article started popping up online. The message-board debates, as many online do, were levelheaded at first, then devolved into the ridiculous and vitriolic. While the first bunch of comments I read contained sensible criticisms about my methods (feeding Bea meager packs of processed snack foods, snatching a hot chocolate out of her hands at Starbucks), the discussion soon turned into allegations of insanity and abuse, complete with a recommendation that Child Protective Services be called on Bea's behalf.

While I probably shouldn't have been surprised by the maliciousness of the discourse my article generated—this was the Internet age, after all—it felt surprisingly painful to read anonymous attacks on me and my parenting. I snapped my laptop shut. I was not going to read any more. I could be satisfied that my article was being talked about. There was no need to read the venom.

But calls, emails, and texts from my friends made ducking the maelstrom impossible. They were worried about me, checking in to see if I was okay. I learned that bloggers were devoting entire articles to me, and the comments on those articles numbered in the hundreds, most negative.

Just to get a tiny sense of what was going on, I read one such article, on a prominent blog. It was wrenching. I was called, among other things, "abrasive," "irrational," and "truly disgusting." Those are the printable epithets. The moments that had caused me self-doubt—now immortalized in *Vogue*'s pages—were excerpted as clear evidence of my unambiguously awful parenting. My admissions about my teenage food and weight struggles were invoked as proof that I was projecting my own neurotic issues onto Bea. I was accused of having superficial motivations for forcing Bea to be "skinny," and that getting myself a byline and photo in *Vogue* was one of them.

I felt physically sick. I had written an unsparingly honest article that I'd thought people could relate to. But apparently I had inadvertently outed myself as a selfish, cruel mother. It wasn't as if I had been misrepresented or misquoted. *I had written the article myself.* Those were my own words. And virtually everyone who read them seemed convinced I was despicable.

According to friends monitoring the situation, our nutrition doctor was being widely quoted in response to my article. She'd told the blog *Jezebel* that she "wasn't thrilled" with the way my piece in *Vogue* depicted her program. She criticized me for ignoring the "emotional issues" involved, and disclosed that I had given up on our appointments after a few months. She conjectured that, had we stayed under her care, "the end result would have been more than just weight loss: [we]'d have weight loss and a happy child."

I understood that she kind of had to throw me under the bus, lest the tsunami of anger cast her as an accessory to the crime. Still, I wasn't sure why she needed to conjecture about the emotional well-being of a child she had personally treated only a handful of times and hadn't seen in over a year. But most of her remarks seemed to just be setting the record straight about the tenets of her program.

When Jeff read some of the coverage, he shrugged it off. "It's just some stupid bloggers," he said. "Who cares?"

I knew he was being intentionally flippant. When you're married to someone as prone to stress and self-flagellation as I am, it helps to act as though things are no big deal, to try to ratchet down the emotional response level a few notches. It meant an enormous amount that Jeff was on my side when external voices were so resoundingly against me. He remained so even when we had to scramble to remove all online traces of our kids after a British tabloid published a photo of our family that they'd pulled off his Facebook page.

"You know why you're doing this, and we've talked about it," he reminded me in the middle of the night, when I couldn't sleep from all the stress. "This is for Bea. You know what you've achieved together, who she is, and who you are. That's what you have to hold on to."

But these bloggers, and the chorus of commentators who had not necessarily read the full text of my article, were confirming my worst fears throughout this process: I was crazy, and now I had made my daughter crazy. Food, dieting, and weight were eternal struggles for me, and now they would be for her. While I had naively hoped I could get beyond my own baggage and help Bea get healthy, doing so had backfired, and now I had screwed her up for life. She would have been better off if I had left her alone—or if she had had a better, issue-free mother to shepherd her through the process.

Jeff, reassured me that we'd done the right thing, and that while people could say what they wanted, they were not fit to judge unless they knew us, knew Bea, or had successfully ushered their own obese children into health while preserving their self-esteem and happiness.

He'd have to have similar conversations with me many times over the next few days as I processed what was going on. He'd remind me that Bea was a very happy child. He pointed out that one of the major reasons I'd written my article was to address the very kinds of reactions that the article was getting: attacks on a regular person trying her best to deal with the colossal challenge of helping an obese child lose weight.

Most of all, he felt that what people were responding to was not even a weight issue but a parenting issue. People did not want to accept the possibility that a good mother could publicly admit to the bad parenting moments I'd laid bare without being crucified.

Everyone had acted the way I did at one time or another, he said. Few are willing to confess to it. And my doing so had struck a nerve at least as great as one about food and weight and little girls.

We all want to do what's best for our offspring, but that means different things for different children, and to different parents. Do we want to maximize our kids' joy? Keep them as safe as possible? Push them as hard as we can to help them reach their fullest potential? No matter how far you're willing to go for your child, you can't give them everything. As the response to my article had clearly illustrated, one's definition of what's "best" is inevitably going to run counter to someone else's.

Over the next few days, the response to my article intensified as media outlets picked up on the online backlash. My home answering machine filled up with messages from CNN, *People,* the *Toronto Star,* Headline News, Dr. Phil, Dr. Drew, *Showbiz Tonight,* even the *Times* of London.

One of the few calls I took was from one of my aunts. She is a brilliant woman, a successful doctor, a devoted wife, and mother to three grown children. She is fun and interesting and funny. She is also brutally honest with everyone, sometimes to the point of insult. She cannot go shopping or even attend one of her grandchildren's birthday parties without getting into an argument with somebody.

She harangued her children throughout their childhoods in the interest of pushing them to be the best they could be. In one infamous incident, she so badgered her middle child in the waiting room of a doctor's office that a stranger passed the child a note with a phone number, offering help if she wanted to escape (I'm not telling tales out of school; my aunt will recount this story with a laugh).

But anyone who would, based on casual observation, consider

my aunt to be a bad mother would be utterly wrong. She gave her kids such vast stores of unconditional love, respect, and support that none of them ever doubted her absolute—and often embarrassing—adoration, coupled though it sometimes was with yelling. All three of her children grew to be happy, healthy, and successful. They are sensitive, kind adults with great families of their own, and, for the record, they could not love their mother more.

I love her, too. Because even though she would vocally critique my appearance, disapprove of my boyfriends, or belittle my professional endeavors if that was how she saw things, she was doing it only because she thought I'd benefit from hearing her opinions. She'd also be the loudest in her praise when she felt I looked great, had met the right guy, or was doing well at work. And I never doubted that she loved me or wanted the best for me.

She called me that day to tell me I had to be more like her.

"Don't listen to anyone," she said. "You did the right thing. You have to be like me—just be confident no matter what. Because you know that your kids are the best and they're happy. No one can tell you otherwise."

I don't share my aunt's natural assurance or moxie, but in that moment (and in many more since) I wished that I did. Because while it was easy for others to look at what I wrote and paint me as an abrasive, cold, superficial person, I felt my actions were being misunderstood. Still, being a public villain is not an enviable ride. And I wanted the controversy to just go away.

I realized, too late, that by appearing in *Vogue,* I had unwittingly presented myself as some kind of fancy Manhattan mom. That erroneous supposition was picked up and promulgated on the Internet until even legitimate media outlets described me as "socialite Dara-Lynn Weiss," as though it were just a plain fact.

It shouldn't have mattered, but I think it affected how people responded to my article. They viewed me as an unrelatable society woman whose life and decisions were nothing like their own. It made my story easier to process. By avoiding the mundane reality of the situation, they didn't have to confront the question of what they would do in my position.

On the other hand, maybe I'm not giving my critics enough credit. Perhaps they didn't care who I was or what my motivations were. I knew from personal experience that to many people, the idea of putting a child on a strict diet and unyieldingly keeping her on it was abhorrent. It didn't matter what kind of person I was; doing what I did made me a bad mother.

I also woke up to the fact that *Vogue* is not *Parade* magazine. *Vogue* is a periodical that is—as *The New York Times* described it in an article about my essay—"possibly the spiritual home of the eating disorder." I'd underestimated how powerful and, to some women, dangerous that particular venue was for my particular story.

The support of my friends, family, and especially Jeff helped give me clarity amid the craziness. They gave me the courage to act around Bea and David as though everything were normal. While I was deeply shaken, I didn't want the kids to know about it. When they overheard conversations I was having about the backlash and asked what was going on, I blandly explained that some woman wrote an article about my article and said that she thought I was too tough on Bea. We hoped we could leave it at that.

I was terrified, though, that the controversy had already grown too big and that Bea was going to be the target of comments at school. We'd have to wait until she went back the following Monday to find out. I berated myself for failing to heed the advice to leave Bea out of the photo. I felt stupid for not thinking of using a fake name for myself. If only I hadn't been so naive about the potential reaction!

In the meantime, I couldn't entirely avoid the headlines. I received an email inviting me to my friend's new baby's bris, and at the bottom, fed in through some Yahoo! News technology, was a link to an article: "A woman uses dramatic methods to get her seven-year-old to lose weight before a magazine photo shoot." Ugh.

A later Google search revealed a smattering of articles in my defense, including ones on sites as prominent as *Time* magazine's *Ideas* blog and Fox News. But of course, these supporters were drowned out by my critics. More than 100 articles had been written about my essay, hundreds more blogs had posted about those articles, and those presumably generated thousands of reader comments.

I don't say proudly that the online controversy was of international proportions. Articles were written about me in Poland, India, Italy, France, England, Canada, Germany, Lithuania, Brazil, Ireland, Australia, and Hong Kong, and they all agreed I was pretty disgusting. I don't know German, but I can take a guess as to what the headline "Monster-Mutter No. 1" means.

But people who were actually touched by this problem personally went out of their way to contact me to express their support. Women and men who have struggled with their weight all their lives commended me for getting involved with Bea's problem early. People with siblings who battled eating disorders shared their suspicion that the situation might have been avoided if their parents had been willing to talk about weight. Several mothers of overweight adults told me their grown-up children blame them for letting them grow up fat and not doing anything about it. A woman with a young overweight child confided that she identified with my feelings of awkwardness and being judged in dealing with the issue.

Those conversations were the most reassuring to me, because these were the people who had lived this problem, not just judged it from afar.

My journey had been beset by doubts, and the backlash to my article had reinforced those fears. But I slowly began to think that, just maybe, I had done the right thing after all. The more closely I considered the criticisms against me, the less validity I felt they had.

The harshest allegations were that I "fat-shamed" and "publicly humiliated" Bea. I recoiled from the accusation but struggled to understand what people were referring to. When exactly did I fat-shame and publicly humiliate her? By getting testy about the hot chocolate at Starbucks? Was it the enforcement of her dietary restrictions in public? What about all the parents of healthy-weight kids who do that? Are they exempt from censure because their kids aren't fat? Did any policing of Bea's food intake become "public humiliation" just because the result I was seeking was not just instilling generally good eating habits but managing her weight?

Maybe if Bea hadn't been lying on her stomach in one *Vogue* shot and obscured by a table in the other, people would have realized that the goal I achieved was not to make her "skinny" or "slender" or "thin," which is how various journalists described her, although those words do not appear once in my article. In fact, at both the time of the article's writing and its publication, she was still technically in the "overweight" category. Does that make people feel better?

Some friends ventured that perhaps my own weight affected how readers viewed my plight. That maybe some readers inferred I was disappointed that my daughter didn't look like me. Perhaps if I'd been visibly overweight or discussed my husband's family history with obesity in greater detail, I would have appeared more sympathetic. Or in that case would my insistence on seeing to it that Bea didn't end up like us seem hypocritical? I could easily imagine being excoriated for forcing my daughter to lose weight while allowing myself or my husband to be heavy. But the converse didn't seem to satisfy people, either.

Another major source of rancor was that I went public with our story at all. People felt that my writing about Bea's weight was embarrassing to her. This is a private issue, they railed, and should have remained so. To me, such concerns reveal a misunderstanding of how inherently public it is to deal with being overweight. Obesity is an excruciatingly obvious disease. Having fought her way to a healthy weight, I'm not sure what these critics believed Bea should feel embarrassed about.

My favorite criticism was that I vocally disapproved of her food choices and refused her food even when she complained of being hungry. Are you kidding me? Of course I did that! When more exercise and a healthy diet fail to make a difference, how else can one address obesity other than by reducing an overeater's food intake?

Finally, just about every critic used one or more of the following adjectives to describe me: "tone-deaf," "obsessive," "strict," "abrasive." And to those critics, I say: guilty as charged.

But that doesn't mean what I put Bea through was cruel or wrong. What if the difference between me and the millions of mothers who haven't yet curbed their children's obesity is the very actions that people were so shocked by: the inflexibility, the harshness? Well, you could argue that in that case, I should have let her be. Fighting a child's obesity is not worth making her miserable. Health is not just about the body, it's also about the mind.

But the fact remains that I really do not believe that aborting Bea's consumption of hot chocolate at Starbucks, having an annoying conversation about dessert at every party, making her enumerate her snacks at French Heritage Day, and refusing her a fifth piece of fruit before bed have made her life unbearable. I bet she would agree.

I was on edge as I drove the kids to school on their first day back after everything blew up. What if I had a car accident? I imagined the blog headline: "God Delivers Justice for Bea: *Vogue*'s Diet Mom Dead in Car Wreck."

I was preoccupied all day, wondering what she was going through at school. I waited nervously at her bus stop for her in the afternoon. When she arrived and climbed off the bus, I scanned her face for any sign of what her day had been like. Had any kids made comments? Mentioned the article? Tipped her off to the backlash against her mom?

She reached the street, dragging her wheeled backpack behind her. She opened her mouth and uttered the two familiar words she always said when she got off the bus: "I'm hungry!"

I had never been so happy to hear it.

CHAPTER 23

If Scarlett Johansson's beautiful face looked especially lovely smiling out at me from the May issue of *Vogue*, it was likely because the image confirmed that the issue containing my article was no longer on the newsstands.

It had been a difficult month being the hated *Vogue* diet mom. I was glad that the controversy had finally died down and that my kids had emerged as buoyant as ever, reasonably unaware of the controversy their mommy had unwittingly sparked.

But the outcry had affected me. The disapproval, scorn, and fury unleashed in response to my article reminded me of the real proportion of supportive voices versus critical ones and revealed the true tenor of society's response to what I did. The world had more clearly exposed its inability to deal unemotionally with the intersection of weight, food, children, obesity, and parenting than I ever could have. My complex and multidimensional story had been reduced to the tale of a cruel, narcissistic mother who shamed and tortured her daughter into socially acceptable thinness, handing her an eating disorder along the way.

So many outside observers had refused to accept any nuance, elided my humble admissions of ill-preparedness and uncertainty, and jumped to flawed conclusions to fill in any blanks left by my article. In doing so, they demonstrated how their own narrow notions affected their interpretation of my words and actions. To them, a candid acknowledgment of obesity equates with shame. Public discussion about how to feed an overweight child is public humiliation. Denying food to an overweight child is deprivation, even "starvation." Many of the reproaches revealed an ignorance about obesity. Still more demonstrated an inability to accept that a person can make difficult decisions, be strict, and even make mistakes, yet still be a good, loving mom with a child who ends up physically and emotionally healthy.

I appreciate that the public rushes to judgment to protect a young child, but why did everyone assume that my interactions with her were abusive? If I get testy with a food server, refuse Bea a second dessert, even hold back most of her dinner because she ate too much for snack, those things do not necessarily entail cruelty. They can be, and were, actions taken with love and respect.

Helping an overweight child is hard. Doing so as a woman in today's weight- and food-obsessed culture, as someone who has grappled with her own issues of body image, is even harder. People don't need more excuses to avoid dealing with childhood obesity. I wish the media hadn't provided so many in their response to my story.

Coincidentally, while my *Vogue* article was on newsstands, a relevant controversy erupted in nearby Park Slope, Brooklyn. Apparently some neighborhood parents were in an uproar about the presence of an ice-cream truck at a popular playground. This dust-up began with irate moms posting online, and it eventually received television and print coverage as far away as Seattle and San Francisco. The problem at hand was that there was an ice-cream truck in full view of the kids, and children were freaking out and having "meltdowns" if they were denied ice cream by their caregivers. So some moms wanted the truck banned from the vicinity.

Relieved to see that the media heat had moved on to another target, I observed with interest how blogs and newspapers presented the drama. The gist of the coverage was generally mocking the parents for being unable to countenance conflict with their children. A *New York Observer* reporter wrote, "Rather than teaching kids to deal with temptations and master their impulses, parents would like those temptations removed. Now! Please." And while this story was never overtly connected to the outcry my article ignited, there were some fascinating parallels.

One Park Slope mother complained that she had to fight with her kids every day at the playground over the ice-cream issue. This mom was subjected to media ridicule for her perceived unwillingness to discipline her child. Huh? So now it's a good thing to discipline a child around food? In any event, no one accused her of "publicly shaming" her kid.

Another Park Slope mom opined that parents need to learn how to say no and that kids need to learn how to hear it. She was presented as a reasonable voice, not as someone "depriving" her child.

While I felt like an outcast for monitoring my child's food intake and admitting that publicly, a woman who spoke to the *New York Post* requested anonymity "for fear of being ostracized by other parents" because she disagreed with the bloc of parents who wanted the ice-cream trucks banned. Imagine fearing social reprisal for disagreeing with food-policing parents! Where were all the anti-ice-cream moms when my article came out?

I was vaguely amused by the local controversy—which, predictably, petered out after a few days. But on another level, it made me sad that this situation, which, like mine, involved food, kids, and overbearing moms, was received so differently in the realm of public opinion.

I think the disconnect comes from the ever-uncomfortable issue of weight. In the Park Slope ice-cream truck story, none of the kids involved was identified as being overweight. So their parents could feel free to give them ice cream, to say no, or even to go to the extreme of wanting a ban on ice-cream trucks. None was called abusive. If only these parents understood the daily strain of saying no and no and no again while one's adorable, sweet child keeps saying, "Why not?" Of trying to convince one's heavy child that she wasn't really as hungry as she constantly announced, of wanting a daughter to be and *feel* healthy when she wasn't old enough to remember what being lighter and healthier felt like.

I admit that I cannot predict what will happen to Bea in the future. I live with the worry that this experience will somehow hurt her later in life. I of course fear the possibility that she may develop an eating disorder, though it's impossible to predict. Food was not a fraught issue in my household, yet I developed problems with it. My two sisters, who grew up in the same environment, did not. Bea and her brother, just one year apart in age and raised in the same home, have vastly differing approaches to food. How do we make sense of that? There is no blueprint for neurosis.

Parental pressure is frequently faulted by people suffering from eating disorders, but so is parental failure to intervene with weight and food issues. It's a lose-lose proposition for parents. But maybe a parent's attitude toward food and weight is not as central to the issue as we think. In 2002, a genetic link was found to eating disorders. One of the researchers stated that as far as the onset of eating disorders goes, "sociocultural factors are only important in that they might elicit an expression of someone's preexisting genetic predisposition."

So we're back to what I asserted at the start: there are some issues that kids are just born with. I didn't make Bea obese. I don't blame sugary drinks, processed foods, trans fat, or gargantuan portion sizes. She didn't become overweight because she gorged on junk food or played video games all day. She was simply and indisputably born with the unfortunate tendency to overeat and a congenital preference for foods that are conducive to weight gain. And she was going to be overweight unless she changed her behavior to run contrary to her natural inclinations.

As for the risk of an eating disorder? There, too, I think that's either in Bea's DNA or not. I hope like crazy that it's not, but only time will tell.

Frankly, I'm far more concerned about the far greater likelihood that Bea will suffer the kinds of nagging concerns about her weight that most girls and women do in our society. I am hopeful that the practical and emotional tools we have helped her develop—not the least of which is a comfort level in discussing weight and food, and knowing what is healthy and appropriate—will be useful to Bea in that area. So my choice to take decisive and dogged action with Bea was fairly easy. I had a chance to make her more healthy and happy. How could I not take it?

I don't pretend that I have figured out the best way to fight childhood obesity. I only did what I thought was best in our specific situation. Even though I stand by the path I took and the map I designed, I believe Bea deserves most of the credit for what she accomplished. At age seven, she accepted an eating regimen that most other kids would have roundly rejected. She had the maturity and foresight to understand that the sacrifices she has to make now have a long-term payoff, and that's not something a parent can take for granted in a child so young. Given that I had to deal with this problem, I'm lucky that I did so with a kid as intelligent and understanding as Bea.

Ultimately, parents of obese children need to make their own decisions about how to approach the issue. When my kids were in preschool, two of their classmates had difficulty with some developmental, cognitive, or behavioral issues, and the school recommended that the parents engage the services of a Special Education Itinerant Teacher (SEIT). Each set of parents struggled with the decision. While both agreed with the school's assessment that there was an issue, only one set of parents agreed that intervention was warranted. The other kid's parents felt the school was overreacting. Maybe the child would just grow out of his problems. Why stigmatize him so early as having special needs?

And while, ideally, the SEIT would help the child progress to classroom independence, there would be a permanent record of the services that would follow the child when he or she applied to kindergarten. The parents noted that it would be considered a strike against him in a competitive admissions environment. They also worried that the other families would view the child differently if his need for extra help was displayed so publicly.

I'm not sure how my husband and I would have responded had we been in those parents' shoes. But whatever decision we made, I hope we would have done it with our child's genuine well-being in mind, without being swayed by the opinions of other parents. Parenting is hard enough without worrying about everyone else's judgment.

One thing is quite clear to me: had I been any less strident, any more flexible, we would have failed to get Bea healthy. Had I not opened my mouth—loudly, on occasion—to intervene when she was eating the wrong thing, or when someone was giving her something they shouldn't, or when she wanted to skip karate, or take a cab when we should walk, I can assure you, Bea would still be overweight. Because, as I've said, those little challenges happen every single day, sometimes every hour! If committing to enforcing healthy habits makes me appear humorless and harsh, then so be it. That is what it takes.

It's not like anyone expects leniency in other areas of children's health and safety. Most parents I know won't start their car until their kids' seatbelts are fastened, period. But somehow, when it comes to eating, our anxiety about our children's feelings overrides our concern for their health.

Bea did not need to lose weight to earn my love. She did not need to lose weight to be beautiful. But she did need to lose weight to be healthy. Once I understood that her weight problem was a disease, I had no choice but to treat it as such. Bea may get heavy again, especially in the coming years when she gains more independence and the responsibility for her eating and weight shifts more completely from me to her. If that happens, I think she'll have the tools to decide how she wants to handle it—or not. Whatever she decides, I hope the world will be understanding. I know I'm going to try to be. I know she'll do her best. But anyone who has battled their weight knows how challenging that can be.

CHAPTER 24

Every time I think our story is done, something new comes along that reminds me it's not: a surprising lesson, an incident that proves an old theory wrong, an unexpected setback. But a series of events that occurred about half a year after Bea had reached her weight goal made me feel that even though we'll never be done, we have been successful.

It was the spring, and we were following the diet in the maintenance mode I've described, working on helping Bea sustain her healthier habits on her own. One day Bea said something about having gained a couple of pounds, which indeed she had. She didn't say she was "fat," just that she was a little heavier than she should be. It was such a different experience to hear her say that than those moments a couple of years ago when she was obese and complained about being fat. The tone of her observation was different. It wasn't redolent of the pain and hopelessness that had characterized her earlier comments. Back then, I hadn't known what to say or do. Now I felt more competent to help.

I asked how the weight gain made her feel.

"I need to lose a couple of pounds," she observed. "Especially since this summer I'm going to camp, where I'm going to be eating lunch in the cafeteria every day. But I'll do it."

"How are you going to do it?" I asked.

"Well, instead of having two meatballs with my pasta at dinner, I can have just one meatball," she suggested as a cute example.

I was extremely gratified by her attitude. There was no self-hatred, no negative judgments. Just a realistic self-assessment, followed by a healthy and well-considered plan for keeping herself on track. It was the kind of acceptance of responsibility for herself that I'd been working toward.

When camp time rolled around, I helped her prepare to face that cafeteria on her own. I requested the lunch menu from the director before camp started. I looked up the calorie content of each item and sat with Bea as we discussed which choices she might make. Baked beans or french fries with her hot dog, but not both. Rice only if the taco comes with a soft tortilla, not a hard shell. With some dry penne and a half-cup measure, I showed her what an appropriate portion size was for the days they'd be having pasta. She independently typed up her own little reference chart and put it in her pocket to bring to camp.

That summer I was really struck by how well Bea had integrated the principles of weight management into her thinking. When I picked her up one day and offered her a frozen fruit bar as a snack, she declined.

"I can't," she said. "We made s'mores at camp."

How far we had come since the days when she would "forget"

to tell me about a treat at school until after she'd eaten her afternoon snack!

Then at the last minute, she decided to spend a few weeks in August at sleepaway camp. The tour we took before signing up filled Jeff and me with dread. We toured the giant cafeteria with its multiple serving stations offering bottomless trays of food. We walked through the canteen where, we were told, the kids were given pizza and ice cream every night. The guide took us past the snack bar where the campers could get food between activities. Bea was going to be totally on her own there.

It seemed too big a jump in responsibility level. I trusted her to handle herself at lunch at a day camp cafeteria when we'd discussed what the choices would be. This sleepaway camp deal was ridiculous. There was a limit to what I could expect. I mean, honestly, if *I* went to this camp for three weeks, I'd come back at least five pounds heavier. Bea was still only eight years old.

But we decided to let her go. Jeff had a recurring nightmare in which Bea returned home ten pounds heavier, and he expressed more concern about what that would mean for me than about how Bea would react.

My initial strategy was every bit as neurotic and control-freakish as you have probably come to expect. Before Bea left home, I spoke with the camp director on the phone, making him unequivocally aware of Bea's situation and of the importance of seeing to it that her nutritional needs were acknowledged and supported while she was at camp. I requested the kitchen send me menus for all meals prior to Bea's arrival so I could look up the calorie information for each dish and recommend correct portion sizes.

I talked to her head counselor in advance and explained that it would be best for a grown-up to accompany Bea on the food line in the cafeteria, to help her make the appropriate choices, based on guidelines I'd email before she got there. I suggested someone keep an eye on her between activities and at canteen, to make sure she didn't exceed the appropriate number of snacks and treats. A counselor should be enlisted to oversee her activity choices, making sure she enrolled in at least one physically active class every day and that she didn't take cooking class too often. I also asked that someone take Bea to weigh in once a week and that the results be emailed to me so I could keep abreast of how she was doing.

You know, basic camp stuff.

In retrospect, what strikes me as most amusing about these demands is not how insane I was in making them but how naive I was in thinking I would get the support I sought. If my experience with Bea had taught me anything, it should have been that families helping children with their weight have to rely on themselves to get the job done. Schools, camps, restaurants, and other parents don't have the time, interest, or motivation to understand and adhere to such carefully outlined plans.

When we arrived at camp to drop Bea off, I was still trying to build the support system that had failed to materialize in advance. I identified a counselor who would be Bea's nutrition buddy. While the nurse was performing the perfunctory lice check on Bea, I inquired about how I'd go about having her weigh in every week. When no one could produce the cafeteria menu, I paid a friendly visit to the kitchen myself and asked for it. Told it wasn't yet ready for distribution, I requested a viewing of the document in progress, and photographed it with my cell phone so I could look up nutrition information back at home.

Believe it or not, Bea was not embarrassed by me. Jeff had told her that her ability to attend camp was contingent upon her taking a new level of responsibility for her eating, and upon accepting whatever help the camp might be able to provide. So she was motivated to be successful. She had decided that should any curious fellow campers inquire why a counselor helped her decide what to eat, she'd tell them that her mom was a little nuts about nutrition. Not that she was on a diet, which was too controversial and emotional a statement to make, or that she had a weight problem, which is something no one would suspect by looking at her. Just that she had a plain old annoying health-conscious mom. Yawn.

We drove home after moving her into her bunk, a lump in my throat. This was the longest period of time we'd ever been apart. I was going to miss that little girl. My daughter. My friend.

That first week, I felt confident that Bea's eating was being carefully monitored and that her choices were being guided by the suggested meals I'd emailed to the camp. I heard from her counselor via email that she was doing well and making good food decisions. The weight she reported to me after the first week was stable. I was promised the next week's menu so that I could provide continued guidance.

But the following week's menu never came. Nor did any subsequent weigh-ins. All communication about her eating ceased. A year earlier, I probably would have called the camp every day to find out what was up, maybe even driven up there to see what was going on. But instead I was relaxed. I had confidence in Bea. I envisioned her walking up to that cafeteria food line and making the right choices. I knew in my mind that she had the tools to eat right, and I felt in my heart that she was using them.

Three weeks later, when we came to get her, we found out the truth. No one had accompanied Bea on the food line, escorted her to the snack bar, or watched her at canteen. No one had shown her the meal suggestions I'd emailed to her counselor, and no one had checked that she'd signed up for some elective that involved physical activity every day. She hadn't even opened the nutrition doctor's booklet she'd brought with her for reference (with a strip of duct tape modestly covering the words "Childhood and Adolescent Weight Management" on the cover).

She had made all her food and activity choices on her own.

On that day we picked her up, we joined her for lunch. I watched from afar as she grabbed a plate and stepped up to the food servers in the cafeteria. I saw her ask for one piece of chicken and some broccoli. She shook her head to decline the offered bread, rice, and potatoes (*three starches*? Come on, people). At the beverage dispenser, she bypassed the fruit punch, soda, and lemonade and took water.

We sat down to eat. "I didn't know it at first, but they have dessert in the cafeteria every day for lunch *and dinner*," she told me.

"How did you handle it?" I asked.

"I didn't have it every day," she said without regret. "Sometimes I'd ask for like a quarter of a brownie, just to try it." I was bursting with pride. I told her that was a great way of dealing with it.

We stopped by the snack bar later for relief from the sweltering heat. "Have an ice pop, Mom," she suggested. "The little ones only have twenty-five calories." She picked up an apple on her way out.

I asked her how the nightly canteen was. She admitted that she felt jealous that other campers enjoyed pizza and ice cream every night and she only permitted herself to join them twice a week, but she'd survived. She'd come and just dance or hang out and have fruit instead of the other stuff. She'd had fun.

In addition to being in a play and studying circus (you should see her twirl hoops), she had elected to go to the fitness center *every day* to work out, of her own accord. She'd also gone to cooking class, but only once. And she'd done swimming, water sports, jewelry making, tie-dyeing, and everything else she wanted. There had been a voluntary four-kilometer race for charity early one weekend morning, and she'd participated.

Bea had spent three weeks on her own, with more food and more independence than she'd ever had to contend with before. She hadn't gained a single pound.

More than any weight she reached, dress size she achieved, or attitude shift I witnessed, to me this experience was the closest to what I'd be willing to claim as victory. A couple of years earlier, that camp environment would have been a disaster for Bea nutritionally. Now she handled it like a champ. She didn't feel like an outsider or like she was different. She was a regular, healthy kid. A normal kid.

We'd taught her how to eat properly, and she had taken those lessons and made them a part of her life. Isn't that what we parents hope for?

Despite her mature and responsible behavior, Bea is still Bea. She will still shout excitedly at the television when a cheeseburger appears onscreen. Her favorite iPhone app is one in which she can bake digital cookies, decorate them, and eat them with taps of her finger. She asks to stop in one food establishment or another every time we walk anywhere. When I asked her the other day which word in the English language was her favorite, she answered without hesitation that it was *bakery* because she likes "how it sounds and what it is."

She has not lost her love of food, nor the joy she takes in eating it. She just doesn't do it quite as much. She told me recently that she had a dream about ice cream. But in the dream, the ice-cream menu featured calorie counts.

I'm happy to say she still has her belly. The belly she got from me. The belly she used to suck in as she stood in front of the mirror. The belly she still professes to dislike. The belly I love to hug. It's a reminder she isn't "perfect" by the unnatural standards of our culture, as reflected everywhere from *Vogue* to Nickelodeon. It is a delicious, sweet, evolving symbol of her struggle and her determination.

It's also a reminder of the threat she lives with every day. The looming possibility that she could easily become an unhealthy weight again. It's a reminder to me that I still need to protect her. Sometimes that means refusing to let her make a choice that's bad for her. Increasingly it means letting her make her own choices and hoping for the best. I will eventually have to let go. She's given me lots of reasons to believe she'll stay on the right track.

Sure, I fantasize about a future in which an adolescent Bea grows six inches in a year and suddenly becomes effortlessly, permanently slender. I would love for her to grow up not having to think about food, not having to be careful about her weight. But I suspect that's not in the cards. I expect that adorable tummy, like mine, isn't going anywhere.

And yes, when I look at her belly or hug it, part of me wonders whether it will burden her in the future or become irrelevant, if it will grow or shrink. I wonder if I've done my job as a parent or backed off before my responsibility was met. Regardless of the questions, one thing is beyond doubt: I love that part of her. I love all of her. I wrap my arms around her as she lies next to me, tucked into the curve of my body. I grasp her belly in my hands and pull her close.

NOTES

CHAPTER 2

16 **After conducting a study** Cynthia Bulik, "Strange bedfellows: UNC Eating Disorders program, SELF magazine," *Chapel Hill News*. Last modified May 26, 2008, http://www.chapelhillnews.com/2008/05/06/14350/strange-bedfellows-unc-eating.html.

CHAPTER 5

51 **The statistics quantifying the extent** "Childhood obesity facts," Center for Disease Control and Prevention, last updated June 7, 2012, http://www.cdc.gov/healthyyouth/obesity/facts.htm.

51 **When I was a kid** Ibid.

CHAPTER 7

81 **And each tablespoon** "Cool Whip Whipped Topping—Free Ingredients," Kraft, accessed September 12, 2012, http://www.kraftrecipes.com/Products/ProductInfoDisplay.aspx?SiteId=1&Product=4300000288.

82 **Cool Whip Free became** "Mini Fillo Shells: Nutritionals and Ingredients," Athens, accessed September 12, 2012, http://www.athensfoods.com/products/consumerproduct.aspx?id=12.

84 **In the stumbling-across-information-that-will-prove-your-own-hunch department** Madison Park, "Twinkie diet helps nutrition professor lose 27 pounds," CNN, published November 8, 2010, http://www.cnn.com/2010/HEALTH/11/08/twinkie.diet.professor/index.html.

85 **A spokeswoman for the American** Ibid.

85 **Haub also said** Ibid.

86 **She criticized its use** "Fittingly Mad: Cool Whip Free," Fit Sugar, updated July 23, 2012, http://www.fitsugar.com/Fittingly-Mad-Cool-Whip-Free-371970.

86 **She complained that Kraft** Ibid.

86 **As it turns out** "Cool Whip Whipped Topping—Free Ingredients," Kraft, accessed September 12, 2012, http://www.kraftrecipes.com/Products/ProductInfoDisplay.aspx?SiteId=1&Product=4300000288.

86 **According to the Mayo Clinic** Mayo Clinic staff, "Trans fat is double trouble for your heart health," Mayo Clinic, published May 11, 2011, http://www.mayoclinic.com/health/trans-fat/CL00032.

CHAPTER 10

115 **"If we push our bodies"** Herman Pontzer, "Debunking the Hunter-Gatherer Workout," *The New York Times*, published August 24, 2012, http://

www.nytimes.com/2012/08/26/opinion/sunday/debunking-the-hunter-gatherer-workout.html.

115 **"We're getting fat"** Ibid.

117 **My anecdotal evidence** John Cloud, "Why Exercise Won't Make You Thin," *Time,* published August 9, 2009, http://www.time.com/time/magazine/article/0,9171,1914974,00.html.

120 **The Centers for Disease Control** "How much physical activity do children need?," Centers for Disease Control and Prevention, page last updated: November 9, 2011, http://www.cdc.gov/physicalactivity/everyone/guidelines/children.html.

120 **According to a study of third graders** The National Institute of Child Health and Human Development, "Frequency and Intensity of Activity of Third-Grade Children in Physical Education," *Archives of Pediatric and Adolescent Medicine*, February 2003, Vol. 157, No. 2, http://archpedi.jamanetwork.com/article.aspx?articleid=481246.

CHAPTER 12

128 **During that year, the USDA** Al Baker, "Lunch Trays Got Too Lean in City's Fight Against Fat," *The New York Times*, published September 4, 2012, http://www.nytimes.com/2012/09/05/nyregion/calories-in-some-nyc-school-lunches-were-below-federal-requirements.html.

128 **It bears noting that subsequently** Department of Agriculture, Food and Nutrition Service, "Nutrition Standards in the National School Lunch and School Breakfast Programs; Final Rule," *Federal Register*, Vol. 77, No. 17, page 4111, published Thursday, January 26, 2012, http://www.gpo.gov/fdsys/pkg/FR-2012-01-26/pdf/2012-1010.pdf.

CHAPTER 13

139 **As Thomas Frieden** Thomas Frieden, *The Weight of the Nation,* dir. Dan Chaykin, HBO Documentary Films, 2012.

141 **Forty-eight cupcakes** My Fitness Pal, "Calories in Crumbs Bake Shop Classic Vanilla Cupcake (Small)," page last accessed September 12, 2012, http://www.myfitnesspal.com/food/calories/crumbs-bake-shop-classic-vanilla-cupcake-small-14646566.

CHAPTER 14

153 **Of course, McDonald's is famous** "McDonald's USA Nutrition Facts for Popular Menu Items," McDonald's, published December 2010, http://nutrition.mcdonalds.com/getnutrition/nutritionfacts.pdf.

CHAPTER 17

172 **In 1994, an "expert committee"** Ogden, Cynthia L., and Flegal, Katherine M., "Changes In Terminology for Childhood Overweight And Obesity," *National Health Statistics Report,* Number 25, June 25, 2010.

172 **In 2007, another expert committee** Ibid.

172 **They felt that** Ibid.

CHAPTER 22

209 **She'd told the blog** Katie J.M. Baker, "Mom Puts 7-Year-Old on a Diet in the Worst *Vogue* Article Ever," *Jezebel,* published March 22, 2012, http://jezebel.com/5895602/mom-puts-7+year+old-on-a-diet-in-the-worst-vogue-article-ever.

213 **I also woke up to the fact** Julie Bosman, "Tiger Mom, Meet Diet Enforcer," *New York Times,* published March 30, 2012, http://www.nytimes

.com/2012/04/01/fashion/dara-lynn-weiss-to-write-book-on-policing-young-daughters-diet.html.

214 **I don't know German** "Monster-Mutter No. 1," Kurier (Vienna, Austria), p. 15, April 12, 2012, http://kurier.at/archiv/volltext.php?schluessel=EGEEHGWPOWPROWGHAAOATPST&suche=burgenland&suchevonjahr=2012&suchevonmonat=04&suchevontag=12&suchebisjahr=2012&suchebismonat=04&suchebistag=19&step=prev&offset=399&simple=1&suchseite=.

CHAPTER 23

220 **A *New York Observer*** Kim Velsey, "I Scream, You Scream, Park Slope Parents Scream For No More Ice Cream," *The New York Observer,* April 2, 2012, http://observer.com/2012/04/i-scream-you-scream-park-slope-parents-scream-for-no-more-ice-cream/.

220 **While I felt like an** Michael Gartland, "Park Slope parents back ban on ice-cream trucks in Prospect Park to avoid screaming kids," *New York Post,* updated April 1, 2012, http://www.nypost.com/p/news/local/slopers_creamy_river_lcaxb1lj4D0SHqo4f2K3GO.

221 **One of the researchers stated** Tori DeAngelis, "A genetic link to anorexia," *Monitor on Psychology,* March 2002, American Psychology Association, http://www.apa.org/monitor/mar02/genetic.aspx.

ACKNOWLEDGMENTS

The Heavy is my first book. The fact that you are holding in your hands an actual published volume is thanks to the efforts of many talented, intelligent, supportive people who helped me through the process.

Thanks to David Kuhn, Jessie Borkan, and the staff at Kuhn Projects for making this dream come true, and to Grant Ginder for his hard work getting this project off the ground.

Thanks to those who provided information, opinions, or stories that became part of the book: Mary Bing, Carol Blanco, Robin Frank, Milton Heifetz, Kim Martin, Steven Tuber, and Danielle Adler Witchel.

Thanks to the trusted, smart friends who gave me their honest and endlessly helpful insights on the text: Hilary Hatch and Nina Chaudry.

Thanks to Erik Kahn for legal reassurance, the Ballantine art department for the delicious design, Amelia Zalcman for legal vetting, Penny Haynes for production, Priyanka Krishnan for editorial support, Quinne Rogers for online marketing guidance, and Benjamin "Mindy" Dreyer for attending to all the details.

Thanks to Susan Corcoran and Alison Masciovecchio for deftly handling publicity—no small task on this project.

Humble thanks to Libby McGuire for believing in me, for understanding why this book is important, for wanting to publish it even before it became controversial, and for her unwavering support when it did.

A million thanks to Marnie Cochran, who has spoiled me rotten as my editor by not only being great at what she does, but also cool and fun to work with. She has gone above and beyond as an advocate, mentor, and friend. She made my words a book, and me a writer.

Thanks to the various extended family members without whose support and approval I would have lacked the courage to write this book: Bonnie, Norman, Jackie, and Carolyn Weiss, and related spouses and children; Tata and Yossi; Michael and Judith; and the Kaufmann family and its offshoots.

Without Abigail Pogrebin this book would have remained a far-fetched idea in my brain: her steadfast confidence, helpful introductions, assiduous reviewing and editing of my work, and generous allocations of time and love made this project a reality. I am forever grateful for her friendship.

And finally, "thanks" doesn't begin to approach the debt of gratitude I have to my husband and children. Their thoughts, encouragement, love, pride, and laughter are what made this book possible. They are amazing people. I am lucky and honored to call them my family.

ABOUT THE AUTHOR

Dara-Lynn Weiss is a freelance writer and producer of Internet, print, and television content. In April 2012 she wrote about helping her daughter lose weight in *Vogue* magazine's "Up Front" column. She lives with her husband and two children in New York City.

ABOUT THE TYPE

This book was set in Bembo, a typeface based on an old-style Roman face that was used for Cardinal Bembo's tract *De Aetna* in 1495. Bembo was cut by Francisco Griffo in the early sixteenth century. The Lanston Monotype Machine Company of Philadelphia brought the well-proportioned letter forms of Bembo to the United States in the 1930s.